ALZHEIMER
A Canadian Family Resource Guide

ALZHEIMER
A Canadian Family Resource Guide

Myra Schiff • Lori Kociol
with Dr. Donald R. McLachlan

McGraw-Hill Ryerson
Toronto   Montreal

First published in 1989 by
McGraw-Hill Ryerson Limited
330 Progress Avenue
Scarborough, Ontario   M1P 2Z5

ISBN 0-07-549774-3

1 2 3 4 5 6 7 8 G 6 5 4 3 2 1 0 9

Printed and bound in Canada

Cover and text design by Janet Riopelle
Illustration p. 8 by Julia Hall

Canadian Cataloguing in Publication Data

Kociol, Lori.
   Alzheimer : a Canadian family resource guide

ISBN 0-07-549774-3

1. Alzheimer Disease. 2. Alzheimer Disease – Patients – Care – Canada.
3. Alzheimer Disease – Patients – Services for – Canada. I. Schiff, Myra, date.
II. Title.

RC523.K62 1989   616.89'83   C89-093545-9

This book is dedicated to people with Alzheimer Disease and to their caregivers.

CONTENTS

❧

CHAPTER 8

COPING SKILLS: HOW TO STAY ON TOP   92

CHAPTER 9

DAILY CARE ROUTINES   103

CHAPTER 10

DIFFICULT BEHAVIOURS   114

CHAPTER 11

SPECIAL PROBLEMS   124

PREFACE

Over the years, we have met, talked with, and listened to many people who are caring for family members with Alzheimer Disease and have been impressed by their spirit, patience, and courage. We have observed that they have many skills and have used these skills to give quality care to their family member. We have also witnessed their willingness to share their practical knowledge with others. Several have taken part in family support groups run by the Alzheimer Society and other community groups.

We consider the development of this book to be a step in the sharing process and are sharing our own knowledge of the needs of caregivers. As such, we are serving as a conduit for the knowledge of caregivers from whom we continue to learn so much.

We have striven to provide a practical book that deals with issues facing every caregiver and that supplies information concerning

- what community resources are available and how you can access them;
- what will happen to you and how will you feel;
- what problems you will face, and what approaches you can take to deal with them;
- what choices are available and how you can decide which is the best option.

We bring to this book a set of values and beliefs about people with Alzheimer Disease that motivated us to write it, and we hope they are evident throughout. The most obvious of these beliefs and values is that even though Alzheimer Disease is incurable at the present time, there are things you can do to improve the quality of life for people coping with it. Even if your family member no longer remembers moments of past pleasure, they will have meaning for him or her while they are happening.

Fundamental to our approach is the conviction that people with Alzheimer Disease should be treated with dignity. This means that, regardless of the level of their intellectual functioning, we must assume that their feelings are intact and that they understand and respond to the way other people relate to them. Since at any given moment we will never know how much a person understands, we should always treat that person as if he or she understands everything. Treating a person with dignity also means believing that the type of residence, the treatment, and the care received do make a difference. It also means not talking about them in the third person when they are present, and behaving toward them in a way that helps them maintain their self-esteem and their sense of self-worth.

Another basic belief is that the behaviour of people with Alzheimer Disease is meaningful, if only we were able to understand the context within which they are operating. Their behaviour is purposeful within their own minds, although they lack the skills to act on their intent in a conventional way.

It is essential to focus on people's strengths and their remaining abilities, rather than on their weaknesses and what they have lost. This will make life more pleasurable for you and less frustrating for the Alzheimer patient.

In addition to our concepts about people with Alzheimer Disease, we also hold some important basic beliefs about their caregivers. We believe that you as the caregiver are an active member of the caregiving team and, as such, have rights as well as responsibilities. Your constant contact with your family member gives you valuable insights into how to provide the best care. As a result, you should be listened to by the other members of the care team.

The caregiver has the right and responsibility to look after his or her own interests, as well as those of the person to whom care is provided. If you become overtired or excessively stressed, you cannot give quality care; if you burn out or become physically sick, you cannot give care at all.

You are a person as well as a caregiver and you have a right to balance your own needs against those of your family member. This is not a question of neglecting or abandoning your family member but of finding ways to meet your own personal needs at the same time that you provide good care.

The ideas, suggestions, and recommendations in this book have assisted many people who are caring for family members, but they are only meant as a starting point. People and families are different, and what works for other people may not work for you. You should feel comfortable and confident about adapting the ideas in this book to make them work better. Then you, too, will be contributing to our understanding of how to improve the quality of life for people with Alzheimer Disease and for their caregivers.

L.K.
M.S.
February 1989

ACKNOWLEDGMENTS

First, we would like to thank all the family members, friends, and relatives who shared their anecdotes, experiences, and wisdom with us. We could not have written this book without their contributions. Special thanks go to Jim Fisher, Gilda Freeman, Bruce Hodge, Angela Morris, Julie Morris, Charlie Rose, and Myra Wiener.

We also learned a great deal from some valuable publications. No work on caring for people with Alzheimer Disease could fail to acknowledge *The Thirty-Six Hour Day* by Nancy Mace and Peter Rabins. A number of pamphlets and publications by ADRDA and the Alzheimer Society of Canada were also extremely useful.

Thanks to our legal adviser, Kenneth Cohen, for his assistance with the chapter on legal issues and to Avril Lewis for her insights and suggestions concerning respite care in the home based on her experience as respite director at a community agency.

We are indebted to Dr. Irene Campbell-Taylor, speech pathologist at Baycrest Centre for Geriatric Care, for sharing with us her professional research and expertise in communication and Alzheimer Disease. We would also like to acknowledge the assistance of Dr. Lewis E. Tauber, clinical psychologist, for contributing to our understanding of the impact of Alzheimer Disease on caregivers.

Thanks also to the numerous professional colleagues who provided ideas and insights. Special thanks go to Dr. Maureen Gorman, Carol Silverman, Pauline Sackin, Kathleen Francey, and Evelyn Lazare.

Special mention must go to Sandi Armel for her dedicated research work and her unfailing patience and cheerfulness. Her attention to detail and her ability to keep us on track played a significant role in the successful completion of this book.

Finally, thanks to our families and close friends for their support and encouragement and for believing in us and the book. Special thanks to Gertrude Schiff and to the Dessau family.

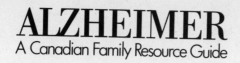

ALZHEIMER
A Canadian Family Resource Guide

1

LEARNING ABOUT
ALZHEIMER DISEASE

❦

T he first time I attended a meeting about Alzheimer Disease, I was floored. I expected that there would be some things I wouldn't understand in the lecture by a leading researcher. What threw me was the discussion period that followed. Everyone seemed to take for granted certain words and concepts I had never heard of. If the friend who brought me had not translated for me, I would have been completely lost.

As a caregiver, you will have many questions about Alzheimer Disease. In this chapter you will find information on the nature and incidence of Alzheimer Disease; what diseases are related to it; and how it differs from other related conditions.

You will need a basic understanding of terms used in books, in lectures you attend, and in discussions with professionals. This chapter will help you find out what some of these terms mean so that you can speak the language of Alzheimer Disease.

TEST YOUR KNOWLEDGE

ALZHEIMER QUIZ[1]

Alzheimer Disease, named for German neurologist Alois Alzheimer, is much in the news these days. The following questions were given to a cross section of 1500 people older than forty-five in the United States in November 1985.

[1] Adapted from *Psychology Today* (May 1987), p. 89.

Use this quiz to see how much you already know about Alzheimer Disease, and what myths you may be interpreting as fact. To compare your answers with theirs and with the correct answers, turn to the end of this chapter.

	TRUE	FALSE	DON'T KNOW
1. Alzheimer Disease can be contagious.	_____	_____	_____
2. A person will almost certainly get Alzheimer Disease if he or she just lives long enough.	_____	_____	_____
3. Alzheimer Disease is a form of insanity.	_____	_____	_____
4. Alzheimer Disease is a normal part of getting older, like gray hair or wrinkles.	_____	_____	_____
5. There is no cure for Alzheimer Disease at present.	_____	_____	_____
6. A person who has Alzheimer Disease will experience both mental and physical decline.	_____	_____	_____
7. The primary symptom of Alzheimer Disease is memory loss.	_____	_____	_____
8. Among persons older than seventy-five, forgetfulness most likely indicates the beginning of Alzheimer Disease.	_____	_____	_____
9. When the husband or wife of an older person dies, the surviving spouse may suffer from a kind of depression that seems like Alzheimer Disease.	_____	_____	_____
10. Stuttering is an inevitable part of Alzheimer Disease.	_____	_____	_____
11. An older man is more likely to develop Alzheimer Disease than an older woman.	_____	_____	_____
12. Alzheimer Disease is usually fatal.	_____	_____	_____

13. The vast majority of persons suffer- _____ _____ _____
ing from Alzheimer Disease live in
nursing homes.

14. Aluminum has been identified as a _____ _____ _____
significant cause of Alzheimer Dis-
ease.

15. Alzheimer Disease can be diag- _____ _____ _____
nosed by a blood test.

16. Medicine taken for high blood _____ _____ _____
pressure can cause symptoms that
seem like Alzheimer Disease.

ALZHEIMER SYMPTOMS

Alzheimer Disease affects a person's intellect, behaviour, and mood.

In the earliest phase of the illness, you will notice a subtle and slow loss of short-term memory. There will be difficulty remembering recent events. The person may seem more easily irritated, and more readily prone to anger than usual. As well, there may be a reluctance to try anything new, and a resistance to unfamiliar situations.

During the next phases of the illness, forgetfulness increases. The person with Alzheimer Disease shows impaired judgment and reasoning ability.

My husband and I were taking a taxi downtown. He paid the taxi fare as usual. As we were leaving, my husband gave the taxi driver a ten-dollar tip—a tip that was enormously out of proportion to the fare. I realized then that I couldn't rely on his judgment as I had done in the past.

There will be problems with speech and language, and difficulties with physical co-ordination. Wrong words are used for objects; words are invented or misused.

The person with Alzheimer Disease will find it hard to make decisions and plans, and will not be able to reason or calculate well. It may be difficult to follow the thread of a story. Mood and behaviour changes vary from individual to individual and may include suspiciousness, or dependency, or hostility.

As the disease progresses, the person with Alzheimer Disease will need increased supervision and help with daily activities such as eating, dressing, toileting, and bathing.

In the later phases of the disease, there is a much more profound decrease in intellectual functioning and the ability to move and speak. Constant care is required and the ill person shows almost no response to people, surroundings, and activities.

This progression of symptoms is often described as occurring in stages, and these are more fully described in Chapter 12.

LEARNING THE VOCABULARY

Alzheimer Disease is a progressive irreversible disease of the brain that results in dementia. It is an age-related condition for which there is no known cure.

You will often see or hear the words *dementia, senile dementia*, or *senile dementia of the Alzheimer type*, (often abbreviated as SDAT) used in connection with Alzheimer Disease. The different terms can be confusing. Some people are offended or upset when the word dementia is used to describe their family member because to them it implies that their relative is "crazy."

DEMENTIA[2]

Dementia is best thought of as a group of symptoms that accompany certain diseases or conditions and not as a disease by itself. Dementia involves the loss of intellectual functions, as well as changes in mood and behaviour. The person showing signs of dementia will become disoriented, and will have problems with memory, reasoning, and thinking. These intellectual losses will be severe enough to interfere with daily functioning.

Alzheimer Disease is the most common cause of dementia; approximately two-thirds of all people who have dementia have Alzheimer Disease. There are, however, other conditions that cause the symptoms of dementia. Use the following brief guide to other dementia-causing diseases to prepare you for further reading or discussions in which these conditions may appear or be mentioned.

Multi-Infarct Dementia is a mental deterioration that may appear similar to Alzheimer Disease, and is caused by multiple strokes in

[2] "Alzheimer's Disease and Related Disorders: A Description of the Dementias," pamphlet distributed by ADRDA (Alzheimer Disease and Related Disorders Association Inc.) (Chicago, 1987).

the brain. Although this form of dementia is not reversible or curable, recognition of an underlying causal condition, such as high blood pressure, can lead to a treatment that may halt the progression of the disease.

Creutzfeldt-Jakob Disease is a rare brain condition caused by a transmissible infectious agent. The course of this disease progresses very rapidly.

Pick's Disease is a rare brain disease that closely resembles Alzheimer Disease and can be difficult to clinically diagnose.

Some people with *Parkinson's Disease* develop dementia in the later stages of the illness. People suffering from Parkinson's Disease lack dopamine which is necessary in the control of muscle activity by the nervous system. The medication given for this disease improves the symptoms of tremors, slowness, and stiffness, but not the dementia.

You should also be aware that a person suffering from severe *depression* may have difficulty with concentration, and can therefore appear to have a dementia. These symptoms can be reversed with proper treatment.

SENILITY

There is nothing wrong with George. He's just getting old and a little senile.

You may hear people refer to what is happening to your family member as "getting senile" or "senility."

What used to be commonly referred to as senility is now called dementia. We used to think that senility was a normal and inevitable part of the aging process.

We know now that this is not true. We can all think of individuals who have lived to be ninety years and are still bright and active. There are sometimes newspaper stories about famous artists or musicians who are still pursuing their careers at a very old age. On the other hand, there are also people who are diagnosed with Alzheimer Disease at fifty or fifty-five years of age.

The condition that Dr. Alois Alzheimer, a German neurologist and psychiatrist, first reported in 1906 came to be known as presenile dementia because the symptoms occurred in a woman who was fifty-one years old. Now, both presenile dementia and dementia are considered to be the same. Both are different from the symptoms that accompany the normal aging process. Senile dementia of the Alzheimer type, or SDAT, is not another kind of condition but is another way of describing the symptoms of dementia produced by Alzheimer disease.

Thus, Alzheimer Disease is a disease that is separate from aging. The symptoms that it produces, including difficulties with thinking, remembering, reasoning, and speaking, are severe enough to interfere with a person's ability to function independently.

> Yesterday I forgot where I parked my car. I couldn't believe that I could forget something like that. It really upset me. Eventually, I calmed down, remembered the closest exit to my car, and found it. I hope that I'm not getting Alzheimer Disease.

> I am so embarrassed. I forgot the name of someone I have known for ten years at a party last night and couldn't introduce her to the hostess. I think I might have that disease I've been reading about.

These are brief memory lapses that happen to everyone. The information that you forget you eventually remember. Everyone forgets things sometimes, and these kinds of incidents do not mean that you have Alzheimer Disease. You may just be tired or overwhelmed, or you may be experiencing stress. Each of these can result in brief memory lapses. Remember that Alzheimer Disease affects not only the intellect, but also behaviour and mood.

AGING AND MEMORY

There are some memory problems that are associated with normal aging, but these are much different from the memory problems that occur with dementia. The following chart shows how normal memory loss that happens as you get older differs from dementia.

ACTIVITY	PERSON WITH AD	MEMORY LOSS IN NORMAL AGING
forgets	whole experience	parts of an experience
remembers later	rarely	often
follows written/spoken direction	gradually unable	usually able
can use notes/reminders	gradually unable	usually able
able to care for self	gradually unable	usually able

Derived from *Care of the Alzheimer's Patients: A Manual for Nursing Home Staff*, Lisa P. Gwyther. This chart is presented in a pamphlet, "Memory and Aging," Alzheimer Disease and Related Disorders Association, Inc. (Chicago, 1987).

At the beginning of this section on Alzheimer basics we gave a definition of Alzheimer Disease. Below is a brief discussion of some of the terms used in that definition.

Age Related   We have said that Alzheimer Disease is separate from aging, and yet it is called an *age-related* condition. This is because Alzheimer Disease mostly affects people who are middle-aged and over. Alzheimer Disease occurs in about three to five percent of the general population over sixty years of age, and in about twenty percent of the general population over eighty years old.

Progressive   Alzheimer Disease brings a gradual decline of abilities. It can seem to start very slowly and "creep up" over a period of time. It can last anywhere from four to fourteen years with an average of six to eight. Although there is a continuing progression of symptoms, there are sometimes plateaus when the condition appears to remain stable. The length of time of these plateaus varies, but eventually decline of functioning sets in again.

The way that the disease progresses varies. Some people with Alzheimer Disease never show some of the behavioural changes that are described. As well, there is no set schedule for how long one phase lasts and another begins. The progression of the condition has general boundaries with great variations among individuals.

BRAIN CONDITION

Alzheimer Disease is a disease of the brain. You need a basic understanding of what this means when you are listening and talking to professionals, and when you come across research articles that assume you already know the basics. The following are terms and phrases used to describe the changes to the brain that accompany Alzheimer Disease.

1. Brain shrinkage: The brain shrinks in size because of a loss of neurons or nerve cells. This occurs mostly in the areas of the brain responsible for thinking and memory.

2. Enlargement of the ventricles or fluid-filled cavities within the brain.

3. Neurofibrillary tangles. These are twisted tangles within nerve cells of the outer layer of the brain known as the cortex.

4. Senile plaques: abnormal clusters in the brain.

5. Protein deposits in and around the blood vessels of the brain.

6. Loss of brain cells at an above average rate in specific regions

of the brain that are responsible for learning and the establishment of memory patterns.

7. A reduction in levels of choline acetyl transferase: an enzyme or protein that is needed to produce acetylcholine. Acetylcholine is a neurotransmitter, a chemical substance released from nerve endings to transmit impulses to other nerves, which is essential to learning and memory.

The following illustration depicts the changes within the brain of a person who has Alzheimer Disease.

HEALTHY BRAIN   ALZHEIMER BRAIN

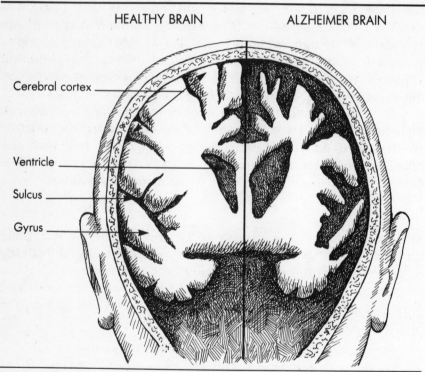

Cerebral cortex

Ventricle

Sulcus

Gyrus

Brain shrinkage (atrophy) is associated with loss of neurons in the cerebral cortex and sub-cortical structures. This results in the decrease in amounts of certain neurotransmitters which function as signal messengers.

We do not know what causes these changes in the brain. As yet there is no cure for this condition, and no way to reverse the progression of Alzheimer Disease once it starts. There may be several factors working together that result in the brain changes and symptoms of Alzheimer Disease. Looking for a cure is an international activity, however, with several research theories being pursued here in Canada.

TRENDS

FAMILY CONNECTIONS

You may have wondered why your family member has Alzheimer Disease when nobody else in your family ever had any problems with dementia.

Heredity may play a slight part in this condition. In one of twenty families there seems to be some family connection–a known relative who has or who had the disease. The role of heredity is hard to determine because sometimes studies have had to rely merely on anecdotal evidence that a relative exhibited the symptoms of Alzheimer Disease. Hence, heredity as a factor is unproven.

Another kind of family connection you may hear about in a lecture or discussion group is sometimes referred to as "familial Alzheimer Disease." This refers to a few families in which there is a very high incidence of Alzheimer Disease. These families are being studied in Canada and the United States to determine if there is an inherited predisposition (tendency to be affected by a particular disease or kind of disease) for Alzheimer Disease. There is a difference in the gene (the basic unit of genetic material) make-up between persons with Alzheimer Disease and their siblings who do not have the disease.

Scientists have observed that nearly all people with Down's syndrome, or Trisomy-21, develop Alzheimer Disease if they live past the age of forty. People with this condition have an extra twenty-first chromosome (one of the threadlike structures in a cell that carries genes).

A PREDISPOSITION IN WOMEN

Women seem to develop Alzheimer Disease about one-and-a-half times as frequently as men. This is probably because women live longer than men.

There is no other "special kind of person" who gets Alzheimer Disease, and no specific Alzheimer personality. People from all professions and work situations, from all economic levels, and from all educational backgrounds get Alzheimer Disease.

MISCONCEPTIONS

With an understanding of this basic information on Alzheimer Disease, you will be able to enlighten people who have false notions about it. These are some of the misconceptions you might hear.

Alzheimer Disease is contagious (there is no evidence that this is true).

Your relative who has Alzheimer Disease isn't really ill and could do better if he or she just tried a little harder.

Your family member is being difficult on purpose and really could behave better in public.

Your family member was always tense and anxious and that's why she or he got the disease.

WHAT IS IT LIKE TO HAVE ALZHEIMER DISEASE?

Reading about Alzheimer Disease and attending meetings and lectures on the subject will help keep you informed, and will help you be a better caregiver. These ways of learning will also help you feel more in control. At the end of each chapter are lists of books, articles, and journals.

Be very cautious when you read reports in the media about "breakthroughs" or new research advances. Always check with your physician before trying out a remedy you read about in a popular magazine. The way the results are described can be misleading, and trying something on your own can be dangerous.

Another way to find out more about Alzheimer is to try to imagine what it is like to have it. Obviously, you can't know *exactly* what it is like. However, the following scenarios should give you some insights into what your family member is going through, and how he or she feels. It is up to you and your imagination to decide how far you want to go with the exercises–the detail you want to get into and the time you want to spend on each of them.

You might also want to share this exercise with other people, to help them understand what is happening to your family member, or you can use these examples to give them some sense of what Alzheimer Disease is about.

Remember that the purpose of this exercise is to give you some appreciation of the Alzheimer person's experience. All of the examples in the list happen to people every day; they were chosen because they are everyday occurrences that are analogous to having Alzheimer Disease. They are not signs of the disease.

1. Think about the last time you lost your car in a parking lot. How did you feel–frightened, angry, bewildered, panicky? Did you feel as though you might never find it? What did you do to find your car? What skills did you use? Imagine how you would have felt if you hadn't had those skills.

2. Remember the last time you locked yourself out of your car or your house. How did you feel? Did you get angry at yourself for "doing something so stupid?" Did other people get angry at you?

3. Have you ever left your house and later were unable to remember whether you turned the stove off? Did you go back to the house to check? Did you call a neighbour to see if everything was all right at the house? Did you do neither of those things, and then worry the whole time you were away? Did you then become obsessive for a while, so that every time you left the house you went back to make sure the stove was turned off?

4. How did you feel the last time you met someone you knew and couldn't remember the person's name? How did you feel when you wanted to make an introduction and could not because you forgot a name?

5. How frustrated did you feel the last time a vending machine didn't work? It wouldn't give you what you wanted and it wouldn't return your money, and nothing you did (kicking, hitting, swearing) made any difference, because things were beyond your control.

6. Think back to when you were part of a group of three or four people who were having a wide-ranging conversation for a half hour or so. Suddenly, someone said "How did we get onto this topic, anyway?" Did the question disturb you?

7. Imagine that you are sitting with a group of old friends. In the middle of the conversation you start to daydream, when suddenly you hear someone saying to you, "What do you think about that?"

8. Have you ever watched a movie with a very complicated plot and you had a lot of difficulty following it? Have you ever

walked into a movie halfway through, or turned on a television show when it was half over, and not known who the characters were or how they related to each other?

9. Did you ever take a vacation in a country where you did not understand the language and you had difficulty communicating with the people around you? Imagine the problem being compounded by the use of a different alphabet, such as Hebrew, Arabic, Greek or Russian.

10. Remember how frustrating it can be to sit in traffic in rush hour and have no control over how fast you can move and when you will get to your destination?

ALZHEIMER QUIZ ANSWERS[3]

	TRUE	FALSE	DON'T KNOW
1. **False.** There is no evidence that Alzheimer Disease is contagious, but given the concern and confusion about AIDS, it is encouraging that nearly everyone knows this fact about Alzheimer Disease.	3%	83%	14%
2. **False.** Alzheimer Disease is associated with old age, but it is a disease and not the inevitable consequence of aging.	9	80	11
3. **False.** Alzheimer is a disease of the brain, but it is not a form of insanity. The fact that most people understand the distinction contrasts with the results of public-opinion studies concerning epilepsy that were done 35 years ago. At that time, almost half of the public thought that epilepsy, another disease of the brain, was a form of insanity.	7	78	15
4. **False.** Again, most of the public knows that Alzheimer Disease is not an inevitable part of aging.	10	77	13

[3] Adapted from *Psychology Today* (May 1987), p. 93.

5. **True.** Despite announcements of "breakthroughs," biomedical research is in the early laboratory and experimental stages and there is no known cure for the disease.   78   8   17

6. **True.** Memory and cognitive decline are characteristic of the earlier stages of Alzheimer Disease, but physical decline follows in the later stages.   74   10   16

7. **True.** Most people know that this is the earliest sign of Alzheimer Disease.   62   19   19

8. **False.** Most people also know that while Alzheimer Disease produces memory loss, memory loss may have some other cause.   16   61   23

9. **True.** This question, like number 8, measures how well people recognize that other problems can mirror Alzheimer symptoms. This is crucial because many of these other problems are treatable. In particular, depression can cause disorientation that looks like Alzheimer Disease.   49   21   30

10. **False.** Stuttering has never been linked to Alzheimer Disease. The question was designed to measure how willing people were to attribute virtually anything to a devastating disease.   12   46   42

11. **False.** Apart from age, research has not uncovered any reliable demographic or ethnic patterns. While there are more older women than men, both sexes are equally likely to get Alzheimer Disease.   15   45   40

12. **True.** Alzheimer Disease produces mental and physical decline that is eventually fatal, although the progression varies greatly among individuals.   40   33   27

13. **False.** The early and middle stages of   37   40   23

the disease usually do not require institutional care. Only a small percentage
of those with the disease live in nursing
homes.

14. **False.** There is no evidence that using   9   25   66
aluminum cooking utensils, pots, or
foil causes Alzheimer Disease, although
aluminum compounds have been
found in the brain tissue of many Alzheimer Disease patients. They may
simply be side effects of the disease.

15. **False.** At present there is no definitive   12   24   64
blood test that can determine with cer-
tainty that a patient has Alzheimer Disease. Accurate diagnosis is possible
only upon autopsy. Recent studies suggest that genetic or blood testing may
be able to identify Alzheimer Disease,
but more research with humans is
needed.

16. **True.** As mentioned earlier, many med-   20   19   61
ical problems have Alzheimer-like
symptoms and most of these other
causes are treatable. Considering how
much medicine older people take, it is
unfortunate that so few people know
that medications such as those used to
treat high blood pressure can cause
these symptoms.

FURTHER READING

Health and Welfare Canada. *Alzheimer Disease: A Family Information Handbook.* March 1984.

Heston, Leonard and White, June. *Dementia: A Practical Guide to Alzheimer's Disease and Related Illnesses.* New York: W.H. Freeman and Company, 1983.

Jorm, A.F. *A Guide to the Understanding of Alzheimer's Disease and Related Disorders.* New York: New York University Press, 1987.

Kra, Siegfried, M.D. *Aging Myths.* New York: McGraw-Hill, 1986.

Ross, Marvin. *The Silent Epidemic: A Comprehensive Guide to Alzheimer's Disease.* Willowdale: Hounslow Press, 1987.

2

THE STAGES OF ALZHEIMER DISEASE: AN OVERVIEW

❧

As a caregiver you will find it helpful to know that Alzheimer Disease generally takes a course through three stages: an early stage, a middle stage, and a late stage.

Throughout these stages, you will encounter changes in a patient's physical condition, intellectual capacity, behaviour and mood, and ability to perform daily tasks. At the same time, there is no distinct line that separates one stage from another. There is no test you can do, or special sign you can watch for, that will tell you that one stage is ending and another is starting. The stages will overlap and merge with one another.

There is also no rule about how long one stage will last. Some people with Alzheimer Disease may seem to remain stable and at the same plateau for a number of years, while others show a much more rapid decline through the stages of the illness. Alzheimer Disease can last anywhere from four to fourteen years with an average of six to eight.

Although there is a generally predictable pattern, not every person with Alzheimer Disease will develop all the possible symptoms in each stage of the disease. For example, your relative may never become aggressive, or wander at night. You may not experience all of the feelings and causes of stress that are outlined in Chapter 7. These behaviours and feelings are described to help you prepare for your role as a caregiver. Adapt the resources in this book to fit your own individual situation.

Differences in the length of stages and kinds of symptoms exhibited may relate partly to the pattern of changes in the brain, partly to the person's pre-Alzheimer personality, and partly to the impact of the environment on the person with Alzheimer Disease.

My husband never showed any signs of violence or aggression but I was constantly worried that this would occur because of descriptions I had read of persons with Alzheimer Disease.

The variability in the course of the disease creates difficulty for the caregiver who may just begin to understand behaviour in one stage when new symptoms appear. As a caregiver, you need to achieve a balance between being prepared–knowing what to expect and what to look for–and being overwhelmed because you expect all of the possible symptoms in each stage of the illness.

Use this discussion of stages and the chart at the end of the chapter and the one in the Appendix as planning guides to help you anticipate the changes you will encounter in the patient, and the actions you will need to take.

EARLY STAGE (STAGE 1)

An Alzheimer patient may show a variety of symptoms in the early stages of the disease. These can include an inability to concentrate, unclear thinking, memory and wordfinding failures, and errors in judgment. You may find that the person makes serious judgment errors in business matters. A person may forget how to use the washing machine, although it is the same machine you have had for years.

First signs are sometimes noticed by family members, and other times they are reported by employers or fellow-workers.

My husband was a minister and he began to have more and more trouble writing sermons. One day he forgot how to turn off the turn signal in the car. Since he had been driving for thirty-five years, I knew something was wrong.

My husband was a bus driver. He began arriving earlier and earlier for work because he couldn't remember what time his shift started.

Often, people who are experiencing the first signs of Alzheimer Disease are aware that something is wrong and try to cover up with jokes and making light of the situation.

Since my wife had always described herself as being absent-minded, it was easy for her to excuse and laugh off memory lapses such as forgetting names of grandchildren and missing appointments. It was only after she became anxious after getting lost on the way home that we were able to persuade her to see a doctor.

You may not have thought of some of the difficulties that an Alzheimer patient experiences because of the subtlety of the memory loss.

My husband went out to the local bakery for rolls. I wasn't worried because the store was familiar and close by, and he was well-known to the sales people. I knew that even if he forgot what to purchase or how much to pay, they would phone me or work it out with me later. But I didn't realize that he would have to negotiate a traffic light to get there, and that he would forget what the stop-lights stood for; that he would forget that red means stop.

My wife was co-operative and when it was suggested that she should wash up for dinner, she would go to the appropriate place. However, she would consistently emerge from the bathroom without having washed. We realized later that she had forgotten what "wash" meant, and so had not been able to carry out this task.

You will not be able to anticipate every occasion in which there is a subtle memory loss, but being aware of the problem may help you understand the person's behaviour and be better prepared. There may be very few physical changes resulting from Alzheimer Disease in the early stage. The person may remain strong and relatively healthy and look the same as usual.

In fact, this may make it difficult for you to explain to relatives and friends what is happening. When they visit, they see their uncle or cousin looking the same as usual. Although he or she may forget their names, or some obvious fact, there may otherwise be no overt symptoms. It is sometimes difficult under these circumstances to explain to others what the disease entails, what planning will have to take place, and what might be expected from them in the future.

This may be especially difficult if you need to involve a relative in helping you obtain power of attorney or in some other legal or financial matter. It may help to:

1. ask your physician to speak to a particular relative;

2. use an ally who knows you, your family, and your relative with Alzheimer Disease to help with communication problems;

3. invite relatives to visit so that they can see the behaviour changes firsthand.

EARLY PLANNING

Although you may be able to carry on with your daily routine without too much difficulty, this is the time to see a lawyer. Some legal and financial actions, such as obtaining power of attorney and reviewing wills and insurance benefits, need to happen in the early stages of the disease, when the person afflicted, is able to understand and participate in the process. This is explained more fully in Chapter 6.

Building a network of support services in your own community will help you later when your family member has increasing difficulty with daily tasks, and when you are no longer able to leave your relative alone. In later stages of the illness, when you need the help, you will have less time and be under more pressure than in the early phases. Look for programs that provide meals, homemaker help, day care, and respite care.

You will have more time in the early stages to attend Alzheimer chapter meetings and learn about what is being offered in your community. As well, you may find out about the best lawyer to use, how to apply for special programs, and whether or not there is a family support group you can join.

Let "important others" know what is happening. Informing neighbours, local storeowners, relatives, and friends about your relative's illness is an important step in building a personal support network. As your family member needs more help, you will be able to call upon the members of your support network to provide relief and assistance.

Take measures to ensure that your family member will not wander from home. If possible, enlist in your neighbourhood Alzheimer registry organized by the police department. The Alzheimer Society will be able to tell you if such a service exists in your community and how to use it. You should also identify your relative with name tags on clothing and an identification bracelet, if possible. Make a comprehensive record to give to police if your family member does wander. Include his height, weight, distinguishing features, and a recent photograph.

Identify those areas in which your house needs to be made safer immediately and note the things that will have to be done in the future. If the work must be done by professionals, call them now. If the work doesn't need to be done yet, at least identify who can do it and approximately what it will cost.

Start to identify suitable long-term care facilities in your geographic area. Although it may seem early, waiting until a facility is needed may not give you enough time to examine places or to put your relative's name on a waiting list.

Planning will be easier when you are under less stress. You will have more time to make phone calls and talk to people when your relative requires less supervision and care.

During this stage and into the middle stages, you should think about whether there are some activities you have always wanted to do with your family member or some issues you may want to discuss. You will feel better later if you express your feelings now about your relationship, your life together, and the love you feel.

MIDDLE STAGE (STAGE 2)

Memory loss, inability to concentrate, judgment errors, and word-finding problems that were characteristic of the early stage of Alzheimer Disease continue to decline and become more extensive in the middle stage. Marked speech and language difficulties appear in this middle stage. Sometimes this change emerges in a year or two, and sometimes it takes quite a bit longer.

The patient may be disoriented in time and place and not be able to remember what he or she ate for breakfast, and yet be able to remember clearly events from the past such as details about his or her past career or war experiences. The patient may still be able to read aloud or repeat words, but arithmetic and other cognitive skills become worse.

You may find that the patient is beginning to show some of the difficult behaviours described in Chapter 10 and requires more supervision and care with daily tasks. Urinary incontinence may be a problem during this stage. Increased disorientation and wandering may pose a safety problem. At this stage it will be important to reduce the amount of stimulation and have a consistent routine as much as possible.

In this stage the disease has a more significant impact on your life, since you will no longer feel comfortable leaving the patient alone.

The difficult part is not knowing what is still intact, what the person can feel, understand, experience, and interpret as the intellectual and behavioural changes progress. There may be no obvious physical changes, and although dementia has increased, the patient may still look quite normal. The appearance of normal health creates problems when a patient wanders, since people in the community may not realize anything is wrong. If the patient is outside without shoes or is wearing inappropriate clothing, then a neighbourhood person has a sign that something is wrong.

LATE STAGE (STAGE 3)

In Stage 3, the dementia becomes profound and communication may consist only of randomly uttered phrases with no apparent meaning. There is increased difficulty with physical movements and the patient will require total assistance with daily self-care including feeding, toileting, and dressing. Seizures may occur during this stage and you should consult with your doctor about them.

There will now be many more pronounced physical symptoms. These will include a stooped posture gradually leading to immobility, and total incontinence. The person with Alzheimer Disease becomes increasingly vulnerable to difficulties such as bronchial pneumonia and heart failure, which eventually lead to death.

Many families report that living with a person who has Alzheimer Disease is like a long grieving process. It is good to prepare yourself as much as possible for the ultimate separation that will occur with the death of your family member.

ANOTHER PERSPECTIVE: SEVEN STAGES

As you become more familiar with issues relating to Alzheimer Disease, you may hear people refer to the seven stages. The seven-stage scale was developed by Dr. Barry Reisberg, and is used primarily by professionals for purposes of assessment and diagnosis.

Dr. Reisberg's research shows that the person with Alzheimer Disease loses abilities in the reverse order that they were first learned. Knowing this may help professionals assess whether or not a person has Alzheimer Disease. For example, if a person was able to handle a sophisticated job, yet was forgetting appointments and major responsibilities, one would, on the basis of Dr. Reisberg's theory, suspect that Alzheimer Disease was not the reason for the memory failure.

The chart of the seven stages is included to give you an understanding of Dr. Reisberg's way of describing Alzheimer Disease.

THE SEVEN STAGES OF ALZHEIMER DISEASE[1]

Stage 1	No cognitive decline	No functional problems
Stage 2	Very mild cognitive decline	Forgets names and location of objects Word-finding difficulties
Stage 3	Mild cognitive decline	Has difficulty travelling to new locations Has difficulty in demanding employment settings
Stage 4	Moderate cognitive decline	Has difficulty with complex tasks (finances; marketing; planning dinner for guests)
Stage 5	Moderately severe cognitive decline	Needs help to choose clothing Needs coaxing to bathe properly
Stage 6	Severe cognitive decline	Needs help putting on clothing Requires assistance in bathing; may have fear of bathing Has decreased ability to handle toileting Is incontinent
Stage 7	Very severe cognitive decline	Has vocabulary of six words Has single word vocabulary Loss of ambulatory ability Loss of ability to sit Loss of ability to smile Stupor and coma

[1] B. Reisberg, S.H. Ferris, and M.J. DeLeon, "Senile Dementia of the Alzheimer Type: Diagnostic and Differential Diagnostic Features with Special Reference to Functional Assessment Staging," *Medicine Illustrated* 3(3), 1987.

FURTHER READING

Newroth, Ann. *Coping with Alzheimer's Disease: A Growing Concern.* Downsview, Ontario: National Institute on Mental Retardation, 1980.

Read, Stephen and Jeffrey L. Cummings. "Alzheimer Disease: Past, Present, and Future." In *Medicine Illustrated*, vol. 3, no. 3, 1987.

3

BREAKING THE NEWS
ABOUT THE ILLNESS

All the time my father was in the hospital being assessed he acted as if he were staying at some luxury hotel. Every once in a while he'd say something like "Vacation's over. It's time to pack my bags and go home," or "I don't like this hotel very much anymore. I think I'll pack and go home." When he finally did go home after the assessment had been completed, he never once asked about why he had been at the hospital, or what was wrong with him, or what the doctors had found, or anything like that. How could I possibly tell him he had Alzheimer Disease when he so clearly didn't want to know?

When my husband and I went to the doctor for his assessment, he made it very clear from the beginning that he wanted to know everything that was going on. He'd always been a "take charge" person, and he handled this the same way he handled everything else in his life. He kept asking the doctors what they were doing and why they were doing it, and what the different tests were for. When the doctor finally gave us the diagnosis of Alzheimer Disease, my husband immediately asked about the prognosis and what would happen to him as the disease progressed. Clearly, there had never been any question about whether or not he would want to know what was wrong with him.

Some families find it difficult to decide what to tell the person diagnosed as having Alzheimer Disease, or even *whether* to tell her or him. There is no easy answer, and the question of whether and how much to tell your family member will depend on many different factors. In this chapter, we will help you decide *whether* and *what* to tell the Alzheimer patient and other people, and how to do this.

The question must be considered in terms of what you and the Alzheimer patient gain by telling the truth about the diagnosis. Among the most important factors to consider are: how your family member has handled similar problems in the past; whether you think the person will *want* to know; and whether he or she will understand your explanations. The benefits to you and other members of your family are additional factors to consider.

INFORMING THE ALZHEIMER PATIENT

Some people may wonder why a discussion of whether to tell a patient of the Alzheimer diagnosis is even included in this book. You may have no doubt that the person has the right to know what is happening, and why. Others will say, perhaps equally adamantly, that they could not possibly explain the diagnosis because the person would not understand, or because she or he would be so upset by the news that it would not be worth whatever is gained by being honest. As the stories at the beginning of the chapter illustrate, both these positions–and others–may be correct, since different approaches are best for different individuals.

In some cases the patient may have already been told of the diagnosis by the family doctor or the specialist. However, you may still have to decide how much to tell your family member about the disease and what is likely to happen, and you may have to make this decision many times. As the disease progresses, the patient is likely to forget the nature of the problem. Eventually, the person may even forget that there is something wrong.

It will be very difficult for you to tell your family member that he or she has a progressive deteriorating neurological disease. The person may be upset about the diagnosis. However some patients find it very reassuring to be told they have Alzheimer Disease, since the only other way they can account for their strange behaviour is that they have some form of mental illness.

> My husband had a senior management job with a large firm. When he first began to show signs of forgetfulness and disorientation, we both put it down to stress and overwork–he'd been working a lot of late nights and weekends to prepare for a major new project. When that was over, we decided to go on vacation, and we both came back rested. But two days after we got back, my husband

couldn't find his car in the parking lot, panicked and called me to come and collect him. As he climbed into my car, he started to cry, and told me he was afraid he was going crazy, and losing his mind. He was really scared.

I calmed him down, and we found his car, but he was afraid to drive home. He really thought he was mentally ill, and was afraid he would do something to himself or someone else. I tried to reassure him, saying that everyone becomes forgetful, and that this wasn't the first time he'd lost the car, but he was really frightened, and said these things were happening more often now. He went on like this for several days, talking about being afraid he was losing his mind, and even telling me what mental hospital he wanted to be placed in. Of course, I made an appointment with the doctor as quickly as I could, and when he told us that he thought my husband had Alzheimer Disease (we had to go to a special clinic for a more accurate diagnosis), you could see the weight lift from my husband's shoulders and he sort of smiled. He knew that if the diagnosis was confirmed we were both in for some terrible times, but he felt relieved to know that he wasn't losing his mind.

Now, when things go wrong, he asks me again the name of his problem, or sometimes he just smiles kind of sheepishly and says "There's that old Alzheimer Disease again." Knowing what was really wrong with him, and being able to put a name to it made him feel a lot better.

Some people really don't want to know what is wrong with them, or they only want to know a little bit. Others want to know everything. If we were to use one phrase to sum up the answer to the question about what and how much to tell your family member, the phrase would be "Take the lead from the Alzheimer patient." The nature of the personality, the person's behaviour in previous situations, and the kinds of questions the patient asks should guide you in your decision making.

The list below contains some descriptions of different people. Judge the characteristics of your family member to help you decide whether or not to explain the Alzheimer Disease diagnosis.

1. Some people are very interested in the details of their lives. They balance their chequebooks monthly, often to the penny. When there is a legal document to be signed, they read it carefully and discuss it with their lawyer before signing. When they pick up their car at the repair shop they will want to know what was wrong, and not simply be reassured that it is working all right now. They are likely to do careful research before

buying a new car or a major appliance. These people are likely to ask questions during the diagnostic test procedures and will ask about the diagnosis and the disease and what will happen to them.

Conversely, some people never question their doctors on the grounds that the doctor knows best. Similarly, they do not balance their bank statements—it's the bank's job to keep track of the money—nor do they question their mechanic. These people may not be interested in knowing what is wrong with them, because they want the doctor to make the correct diagnosis and do what needs to be done to provide good care.

2. Some people have a great need to feel in control of their lives. They dislike it when things are beyond their control and seek to bring everything back under their control. These people not only are likely to want to know about the diagnosis, but are even likely to find it a relief to know what is wrong with them. Once they know they have Alzheimer Disease, they have something to which they can attribute their strange behaviour. While they cannot control their behaviour, at least their problem has a name. Naming something is a degree of control.

3. Some people feel very uncomfortable when things are ambiguous or unclear. They like to have issues resolved, and often find not knowing more stressful than the answer. Often these people will express just these sentiments—"I'd like to know what's going on." "It's the *not knowing* that is getting on my nerves." They are likely to seek a reason for their problems early in the diagnostic process, and should at least be told that there may be a physical reason for their behaviour. Once the diagnosis has been determined, they should be told the nature of the problem, at a level of detail that is consistent with their ability to understand.

My wife said many times that she found it really hard not knowing what was wrong with her—and she had expressed that same idea some years ago when she had dizzy spells. So when the doctor told me she had Alzheimer Disease, I right away told her what the diagnosis was.

How a person has dealt with previous life crises such as a business setback or failure, divorce, or a serious illness—his own or others'—can help guide you about how to proceed. When faced with a serious illness, did the person ask a lot of questions, such as what the test results were; what medication he was on and how it worked and what it would do; what the prognosis was; or, did he hand himself over to the doctor?

Telling your family member she or he has Alzheimer Disease may only mean that you are putting a name to something the person already knows is happening. While people with Alzheimer Disease usually do not complain about memory loss, and in fact struggle to keep up, many of them are aware that something is wrong, particularly when the disease progresses to the point where major problems—a lost car, for example—occur. As well, a patient who has been through a comprehensive battery of diagnostic tests will sense that there must be a reason for a comprehensive testing program.

If an Alzheimer patient asks what is wrong, you should tell the truth, though you must decide which version of the truth to tell and how much. You can say that he or she has the disease, which is the whole truth, or you can say that the doctor found a problem with certain parts of the brain that makes the person forgetful (or whatever the problem is). The latter statement is also the truth, but not the whole truth. The decision as to which approach to use should be based not only on your family member's desire to know, but also on how far the disease has progressed, and therefore how well the person will be able to absorb the information. Tell your family member as much or as little as he wants to know and is able to understand.

> Once the problem had been diagnosed, I told my wife that she had Alzheimer Disease, and that it was caused by little knots of nerves in her brain. But she was too far into the disease to be able to remember the name, or what caused it, so finally I just told her that her brain was changing because she was getting older, and she could understand that for a while.

Whatever you do, do not lie to the patient. The person is almost certainly aware that something isn't right, and saying there is nothing wrong will only add to her or his confusion. Similarly, answer questions directly, in as much or as little detail as seems appropriate. If the person asks what will happen in the future, say that he will find it increasingly more difficult to remember and that other people will have to help more. Talk about how the two of you can work together to devise ways to remind him of all he needs to know.

Even though your family member is ill, he or she has the right to make decisions about his life to the best of his ability, and with the knowledge of his present and future limitations.

My husband had always been fascinated by Japan, and had often said that as soon as he retired, we would go there for a month or two. When we found out he had Alzheimer Disease, he said that he still wanted to go to Japan, but that we'd better go soon. We talked about it, and agreed that instead of travelling on our own, as we'd planned, we'd go on a two-week tour. It worked out fine, and I'm glad he made that decision. I never would have thought we could do it.

If you decide that your family member should be told of the Alzheimer diagnosis, but you don't have the courage to do it yourself, find someone else to do it for you. You could ask the specialist who diagnosed the problem; he is likely to have a lot of experience in telling people they have Alzheimer Disease. Another alternative is your family doctor, or a close relative that your family member trusts. It is important that you be present when the patient is told, so you can reassure her or him.

After a person learns of the diagnosis, he or she will require a lot of emotional support. Reassure the patient that you will stay with her and help her through the difficult times, and that you will need to work together to plan for the future.

Depression is common among people who have Alzheimer Disease. (It is also commonly confused with the disease, which is why a thorough assessment is necessary before a diagnosis can be made.) A certain amount of sadness is to be expected. However, if these feelings persist, or if the person is seriously depressed, you should discuss this with the doctor.

INFORMING CLOSE FAMILY MEMBERS

At some point, other close family members need to be told about the diagnosis of Alzheimer Disease, so they may understand the behaviour of the patient and become part of the caregiving team.

Initially, you may feel reluctant to tell other people about the Alzheimer patient's problem. But they must be told since it is the first step in developing a network of friends and relatives who can provide you with the physical and emotional support you will require during the course of the illness.

There is no shame or stigma to having Alzheimer Disease. It is a disease of the brain with a physical cause and physical changes, just like other diseases treated by the medical profession. Concern about what other people will think of your family member should never be a factor in deciding what to tell them. In fact, telling friends, family members, and neighbours that your family member has a neurological illness can help avoid embarrassment when a patient's behaviour deteriorates. A basic explanation of Alzheimer Disease will help others understand that neither you nor your family member can control this behaviour.

Adult members of the family should be told the nature of the diagnosis and at least something about what the future may bring. Once they have digested this information, you can talk to them about how this will affect their relationship with you and with the family member who has the disease. Explain that the person needs even more love, affection, and help in maintaining self-esteem than before, and ask for their help and support.

How the Alzheimer Disease will affect the practical aspects of your relationships with other people will depend on how far advanced the disease is. The abilities of the patient will change as the disease progresses, and your needs as a caregiver will change along with that. As a result, you may wish to repeat these discussions and negotiations from time to time, as seems appropriate.

In the early stages, the diagnosis of Alzheimer Disease may not have much effect on your relationship with close family members. As the ill person becomes more confused, and as the amount of care required increases, the changes will become more profound and pervasive, and you may wish to look to other members of your family for more support. This is fair enough. However, it is not fair to expect people to be able to read your mind. If you want additional help, you must make this clear to the members of your support network. The more clear and specific you are, the better people will be able to respond.

Blood relatives of the family member–children, siblings and cousins–may express special concern about whether the disease is inherited. You should be prepared to deal with this issue, either by telling them what you know or by directing them to a source such as a book or a person who can answer the question for them.

If you have not told your family member what is wrong, or have not used the term Alzheimer Disease to describe the problem to the patient, be sure to indicate that to the other members of your family, so that they will not accidentally "spill the beans."

INFORMING CHILDREN

In some instances, children will need to be told about your family member's problem. As in the case of the Alzheimer patient, what you tell children and how much you tell them about the illness will depend on what they are able to understand.

You may be tempted to protect your children from unhappiness by not telling them that a parent or grandparent is ill. However, they need to know the truth. Children often have a strong intuitive sense of when something is not right, and what they may imagine in the absence of accurate information may be much worse than the truth.

Young children need to be told only that the family member is sick, and has a disease that sometimes makes him or her forget things or act strangely. It is important to explain to the child that the person cannot help it, and that it is not anyone's fault. You may also want to reassure the child that it is not his fault either. Young children probably will not ask if the disease is catching, but may ask if the family member will die. Although Alzheimer Disease can eventually prove fatal, the time horizons of young children are such that a simple "No" is accurate enough.

Older children are able to comprehend more complex information, and can understand better some of the implications of the disease. Whether or not you use the term Alzheimer Disease is not important. However, you should plan to tell older children a little bit about what will happen in the future, and how it may affect them. Be sensitive to their concerns and worries, and let them know that you are willing to answer their questions. Their worries may be practical: If Daddy is sick and can't work, what will we do for money? The children may need to be reassured that you will still be able to take care of them even though you also need to take care of the ill person.

Like other family members, children may have unfinished business with their parent or grandparent, and they have the right to know this business needs to be completed before it is too late.

Some older children may be willing or even eager to help care for the patient, and you should allow them to do as much as they are capable of. Even young children may want to help. They may enjoy just keeping the patient company, and should be permitted to visit as long as they feel comfortable doing so. Their visits may be therapeutic to the older person, especially since children are very often patient, compassionate, and understanding with people they love.

As the disease progresses and the patient's behaviour becomes more extreme, you may need to reassure the children that they are not the cause, and that they are not making the person worse. You may also need to remind them that the sick family member still loves them, but that the disease makes it more difficult to show it.

INFORMING FRIENDS

Since a good support network is one of the basic keys to coping with Alzheimer Disease, it is important to explain your family member's illness to your friends.

In the early stages of the disease, the Alzheimer patient will still look the same, since the disease does not affect physical functioning until the middle stages. In addition, people with Alzheimer Disease often show great ingenuity in covering up their problems. In the early stages, especially on a "good" day, friends may have difficulty believing there really is something wrong with an Alzheimer patient.

This disbelief probably is a reflection of their own fears and sadness about the disease. Tell your friends a bit about what the future may be like. Explain to them that if they wish to have quality time with your family member, they should do so now, because later the person will not recognize them or be able to relate to them.

You will need to talk to your friends about how your family member's disease will affect your friendship. They will need to understand that adjustments, first minor, later major, will need to be made to what have been your normal modes of relating. For example, if you and a friend are used to meeting once a week for dinner, you may need, initially, to modify this to a shorter lunch. Later, you may feel uncomfortable leaving the patient at home alone, and you may want your friend to come to your house instead. However, this is where the development of a support team becomes important so that you, the caregiver, can get out and still get what you need.

As the patient's disease progresses and his behaviour becomes more unusual, some of your friends may feel uncomfortable about being with the sick person. They may become frightened or embarrassed by his behaviour. You might be able to forestall their withdrawal by explaining more about the nature of Alzheimer Disease, and how to deal with the behaviour.

INFORMING NEIGHBOURHOOD PEOPLE

As time goes on, you will need to tell more people about your family member's condition, because the person may get lost in the neighbourhood. You should tell neighbours and nearby shopkeepers about Alzheimer Disease and what you want them to do if the sick person seems to be in trouble.

When people are not sure what to do they hesitate to intervene when someone else needs help. By telling people that your family member is sick, you alert them to the person's needs and are giving them permission to offer help. If you want them to take the patient to their home or shop, give them a piece of paper with your name and a phone number on it.

INFORMING THE EMPLOYER

Except under very unusual circumstances, there is little probability that an Alzheimer patient will be able to continue working after the disease has been diagnosed. If the person owns a business, alone or with other people, the issue of continued employment after a diagnosis of Alzheimer Disease is quite different from those discussed here. See Chapter 6 for a discussion of self-employed people working after an Alzheimer diagnosis.

If you think it may be feasible for the Alzheimer patient to continue to work, you should discuss the option with him. If the person cannot discuss this, then it is unrealistic to think he would be able to continue in his job.

First find out whether the patient really wants to keep working. In discussing this issue, you must recognize that continuing to work involves more skills than simply the job itself. The person must go to and from work without getting lost; must be able to relate to other people; must be able to adapt to changes in routine; and even deal with such mundane matters as lunches and coffee breaks. Even the simplest activity can become complex when a person does not have the usual capacities available. The likelihood that an Alzheimer patient can continue working for very long is quite remote.

However, if together you decide that the ill person can continue working, the two of you and the employer should meet to discuss the options realistically. Explain why you think the person can carry on a job for a time. Explain also the nature of the disease, the way it progresses, the fact that certain skills are retained for longer periods of time, etc. You may also want to discuss how staff could monitor your family member's work, or how his or her job could be adapted to make the work manageable.

The lack of a job may cause anxiety for an Alzheimer patient. Even among the well elderly, who have planned their retirement long in advance, there are adjustments to be made. Your family member may become concerned about money, and without a job, there is lots of time to fill.

In the early stages of the disease, the patient might be able to take on some volunteer work. If you are involved as a volunteer somewhere, perhaps the person could accompany you; or perhaps he or she could be trained to do another task for the same agency, so that you can both do your volunteer work together. Alternatively, you may find a volunteer task that your family member can do at home, such as folding letters and stuffing envelopes.

FURTHER READING

Cohen, Donna & Eisdorfer, Carl. *The Loss of Self: A Family Resource for the Care of Alzheimer's Disease and Related Disorders*. New York: W.W. Norton & Company, 1986.

Muir Gray, J.A. and McKenzie, Heather. *Caring for Older People*. England: Penguin Books, 1986.

4

PROFESSIONAL HELP

❦

Because Alzheimer Disease is a complex condition, you will probably deal with a number of people from the health and helping professions during the course of your family member's illness. These may include doctors, nurses, social workers, and occupational therapists. Even though the credentials of these people may be intimidating, the family caregiver is the most important member of the care team. After all, you know the Alzheimer patient better than the professionals, and you have the responsibility for the patient on a daily basis.

The purpose of this chapter is to help you become an educated consumer of the health services that are available to you, and to help you become an active and important member of the care team.

DIFFERENT PROFESSIONAL ROLES

Before we begin to discuss how you will be working with other professionals, you need to know who these people are and what their roles might be.

Doctors It is likely that you will work with at least two different doctors over the course of your family member's illness. One of these will be a specialist who is especially knowledgeable about diagnosing and treating Alzheimer Disease. As well, you will likely continue to take the Alzheimer patient to the family doctor for various problems. Other specialists may also need to be consulted.

Nurses In some communities there are nurses who have the job of assisting to care for patients at home, including those with Alzheimer Disease. Sometimes these nurses are part of a program specifically for Alzheimer patients. These nurses are trained to help you learn to care for your family member and meet his or her needs.

Social Workers You may encounter social workers in several different capacities. Many community agencies use social workers to carry out the initial interview with someone who is applying for a service, such as a day-care program or a visiting homemaker. If you decide to move an Alzheimer patient to a long-term care setting, a social worker may be helpful in evaluating the setting and assessing the needs of the patient. A social worker may also be helpful for sorting through some of the feelings and problems you experience as a result of your family member's illness.

Occupational Therapist An occupational therapist assesses and works with people who have physical, emotional, or social disabilities in order to increase their ability to function independently alone, at work, and in leisure activities. You may find an occupational therapist on the team that carries out the initial assessment. An occupational therapist may also be able to give you advice on how to help your family member maintain some of his abilities.

Other sections of this book will discuss in more detail the role of nurses, social workers, and occupational therapists in helping you manage your family member's illness. In the remainder of this chapter, the focus is on the role of the doctor in this illness, and how you can work with doctors to ensure that your relative gets the best medical care possible.

YOUR FAMILY DOCTOR

THE FIRST CONSULTATION

When you first notice symptoms that might indicate Alzheimer Disease, you should suggest that your family member go to the doctor for a check-up. (You may want to mention the nature of the behaviour that is of concern, without specifically using the words Alzheimer Disease.) If the person resists, suggest another less threatening and more common reason for a doctor's visit–to talk about another problem such as headaches or stomach upset, or to have the heart or blood pressure checked. Alert the doctor about your concerns before the person goes for this appointment.

If your family member expresses concerns about changes in his or her behaviour before you notice them, reassure the person, and suggest a visit to the doctor to have it checked out. Your calm and accepting manner may help to ease the fear and give him or her the needed encouragement to deal with the problem.

In the course of the check-up, do not let the doctor dismiss the problem as "senility" or as part of growing old. There is no such condition as "senility" and most people grow old without serious deterioration in their mental abilities. Tell your doctor you think your family member may have Alzheimer Disease, and that you would like to be referred to someone who specializes in diagnosing and treating that disease.

If your family doctor makes an immediate diagnosis of Alzheimer Disease based on your brief comments, you should be equally concerned, and also ask for a referral. Alzheimer Disease is difficult to diagnose, and requires extensive tests before an accurate diagnosis can be made.

If your family doctor suggests he would like to do some initial tests before making a referral, you should probably allow him to do so. Many other conditions may cause the same symptoms, and the doctor may have some ideas about other possible causes.

If the family doctor has known the patient for a long time, the doctor may be able to pinpoint an alternative explanation quickly. This will save you and your relative the time and trouble of going through an extensive battery of diagnostic tests, and will also save costs to the health care system.

If the condition does not improve following diagnosis and treatment, you should ask for a referral to a doctor who specializes in diagnosing and treating Alzheimer Disease. It is possible that your family member has Alzheimer Disease along with another problem masking the Alzheimer diagnosis, so that the diagnosis is correct as far as it has gone, but is only partially complete. For example, it is not uncommon to find depression and Alzheimer Disease in the same patient. If your doctor successfully diagnoses and treats the depression, the symptoms may only partially improve, because the Alzheimer Disease has not been identified and dealt with.

Ironically, in the early and middle stages of Alzheimer Disease, the patient is often in otherwise excellent health. Many patients appear hale and hearty, and their continued activity appears to belie the idea that they are ill.

Nevertheless, there may be other medical problems, not related to Alzheimer Disease, that will occur while your family member has the disease. Some may be long-standing problems diagnosed before the Alzheimer Disease. Others will be diseases common in aging, such as arthritis, that develop independently of Alzheimer

Disease. As well, your family member will be subject to the acute illnesses that can happen to anyone–colds, flu, stomach upsets and other mundane conditions. However, these are often not mundane for the Alzheimer patient when the illness or the medication for the illness adds to the person's confusion. Alzheimer Disease may also aggravate existing conditions–the pacing that is common in Alzheimer Disease, for example, may aggravate an arthritic condition.

FAMILY DOCTORS

Although you need a specialist for the medical care of the Alzheimer patient, there is an important continuing role for your family doctor in maintaining the health of the Alzheimer patient and the other members of the family as well. After all, Alzheimer Disease in one person affects everyone in a family. The perspective that a family doctor brings to a family problem makes him or her an important member of the care team.

Besides consulting your family doctor on on-going health problems unrelated to Alzheimer Disease, you may wish to work with him or her on non-medical issues relating to the effect of the disease on the patient and the other members of the family. For example, because your family doctor knows you, the Alzheimer patient, and the family as a whole, you may wish to talk to him or her about managing behavioural problems presented by Alzheimer Disease.

Furthermore, if the specialist who diagnosed the Alzheimer patient is not located in your community, your family doctor will be more familiar with community resources, and could help you more in finding ways to use these. Of course, because caring for a person with Alzheimer Disease is a strain, you should work closely with your family doctor to ensure your own health bears up under the strain of caregiving.

Once an Alzheimer patient has been diagnosed, you, the primary caregiver, the one dealing with the patient on a day by day basis, will become the most important member of the care team. Your doctor will see the patient occasionally, and usually under a particular set of circumstances. On the other hand, you will see the patient on good days and bad days, in a wide variety of moods and situations, and you will know his or her strengths and abilities and see the change in behaviour better than anyone else. You will be the best person to tell the doctor how the patient is functioning; how the disease is progressing; and how the patient is responding to medication that has been prescribed. You will also be the person to administer medication.

Since you are about to enter into an intensive working relationship with your family doctor, in the beginning you may wish to consider how happy and comfortable you are with her or him. If you have doubts about being able to work with your family doctor, it is better to consider making a change in the beginning rather than in midstream.

CHANGING DOCTORS

What are some of the factors that might lead you to think about changing doctors–either right after diagnosis or at some later time? You might want to review the questions below to determine how comfortable you are about continuing to use your present family doctor.

1. What is your personal relationship with the doctor? Is he or she willing to take time to talk with you and to give you advice? Does he or she respect your own judgment, listen to your feelings and ideas, and treat you as a member of the care team, or does he take the attitude that as a professional he knows what is best?

2. How much confidence do you have in your doctor's abilities? Is he knowledgeable about the problems you bring him? Do you feel she has good diagnostic skills? Are you confident that she keeps up with advances in medicine?

3. Is your doctor available to you in emergencies? Is he willing to talk to you on the phone? Is he willing to talk to other members of the family?

4. Is your doctor willing to work with other members of the care team? Was she willing to refer you to a specialist for the diagnosis, or did she resist or take offense? How does she feel about working with other members of the health and helping professions–nurses, social workers, occupational therapists–who may play a role in helping you manage your family member's behaviour?

If the answers to any of these questions are not clear, you should discuss them with the doctor; after all, if you don't tell him you are unhappy, he can't do anything to make the situation better. If you are still not satisfied after your discussion, here are some steps you can take to find a new doctor.

1. Ask the specialist who has diagnosed your family member's condition whether he can recommend a physician in your community whom you could work with. He may know some family doctors who have more experience in working with people with Alzheimer Disease.

2. You can call the Alzheimer Society or the medical association in your community, for a recommendation of a family doctor.

3. You can speak to other people in your community who have had experience with Alzheimer patients to see whether they have a family doctor to recommend.

Whatever the reason for finding a new doctor, and whatever procedure you use, you should be clear about the qualities you are looking for. You have the right to interview several different doctors, and should not feel hesitant in explaining to each what you are looking for in a doctor before choosing the one you will work with.

After Alzheimer Disease has been diagnosed, meet with your family doctor to review the situation. Since he will be responsible for most of the care your family receives, it is important that he be kept up to date on what is happening in your family. Confirm that he has received a copy of the specialist's report on the patient, and discuss the provisions you have made for your family member.

Find out what suggestions he has and review the available community resources. Even if you do not yet need a particular type of resource, you should identify where you will get that support so that when you are in crisis you do not have to run around dealing with the crisis and trying to find help at the same time. Remember that your doctor may not know about all the resources, but may be able to direct you to the sources of information. This is called networking, an art that you should refine as quickly as possible.

MEDICATIONS AND DRUGS

Some otherwise useful medications may not be appropriate for an Alzheimer patient. They may contain ingredients that will cause hallucinations; contribute to disorientation, confusion, or drowsiness; or interact with drugs which are being prescribed for symptoms of Alzheimer Disease.

You should therefore review the patient's medication with a doctor or pharmacist once the Alzheimer Disease has been diagnosed. Start by preparing a list of the medications your family member is taking, who prescribed them, when and what for. Include those that have been prescribed by the family physician as well as those prescribed by specialists such as a cardiologist, rheumatologist, or internist. Include over-the-counter medications that are taken on a regular basis: antacids; vitamin and mineral supplements; aspirin and other non-prescription drugs. Review the completed list to determine the following:

1. Are any of the drugs no longer necessary, because the problem they were intended to address no longer exists?

2. Are any of the drugs redundant, that is, is your family member taking several drugs that do the same thing?

3. Is there a potential for drug interactions? Does one drug negate the function of another, or does one drug enhance the function of another, thereby reducing the required dosage?

4. Are any of the drugs likely to make worse the symptoms of Alzheimer Disease?

Many pharmacies now keep computerized records of their clients' drugs, which make it easy for them to provide drug counselling with respect to the questions raised above. You may want to find such a pharmacy if the one you are currently using does not provide this service.

Once you have developed this record, you can use it to note reactions to the drugs the Alzheimer patient is taking. Try to be as specific as possible in the notes you keep. For example, instead of simply noting that a medication worked, note that the person has not wandered around at night for three nights. This will make it easier for you to talk to your doctor about whether the medication is helping your family member; whether the dosage should be changed; or whether another medicine should be tried instead.

The medication record you have developed will make it easier for you to work with your doctor, and will help you give your family member better care. You will not have to worry about remembering details when they are written down. The record you have developed will also help you keep track of when your family member should be taking medicines.

Keep the drug record up to date, and use it to keep doctors informed about changes in medication since they last saw the Alzheimer patient.

Many drug stores sell plastic pill containers with separate compartments for each day of the week. At the beginning of the week, you can put all the medicine for a particular day into the compartment for that day, thus saving you the need to organize the pills each day. All medicine–prescription or otherwise–regardless of who it is for, should be kept where your family member cannot get to it, locked up and out of reach. If you can manage childproof caps, and your family member cannot, this is another way to keep medicine out of the reach of the Alzheimer patient.

HANDLING DOCTORS' APPOINTMENTS

In the initial stages of the illness, your family member may readily go with you to a doctor's appointment. If necessary, explain that you and he are going to see Dr. Jones, remind him that he has been to this doctor before, and why. ("We are going for a check up." or "Dr. Jones is going to try to find out why your shoulder hurts.") Tell your family member what to expect at the doctor's. (You will need to talk to the doctor before the appointment to get this information.)

As the disease progresses, your family member may become more reluctant to go to the doctor with you, and may become restless during a wait for the appointment. Try to schedule your appointment for a time when you will not have to wait. When you make the appointment, explain that the patient cannot sit in the waiting room and that you would like the first appointment of the day, or the first one after lunch. This approach should be effective for other kinds of appointments too–the dentist, the hairdresser, or the podiatrist. If it is an emergency, and you cannot wait until such an appointment is free, call the doctor's office just before leaving the house to make sure the doctor will be able to see you at the time your appointment is scheduled.

Eventually, you may need to ask the doctor to make a house call to treat the Alzheimer patient.

SPECIALISTS

As mentioned earlier, the medical problems requiring a doctor during the course of an Alzheimer patient's illness can be divided into two major types. One type are those directly related to the Alzheimer Disease; the other type are those that are more or less independent of the fact that the person has Alzheimer Disease. For health matters relating to Alzheimer Disease you need a specialist.

There are a number of reasons why a specialist is preferable to a family doctor for medical aspects of Alzheimer Disease.

1. Most family doctors will have seen very few cases of Alzheimer Disease. The number of Alzheimer patients is growing, but the overall incidence of the disease is quite low for the population as a whole. Furthermore, until recently, most medical schools devoted little, if any, time or attention to diseases of aging. Thus, most family doctors have little formal training in diagnosing (interpreting specialized tests) and treating Alzheimer Disease.

2. Alzheimer Disease is an extremely difficult disease to diagnose correctly. Since there is no cure, it is extremely important that as accurate a diagnosis as possible be made. You want to be sure your family member does not have another, more easily treatable condition that has been confused with Alzheimer Disease.

3. A great deal of work is currently being done to find a treatment and a cure for Alzheimer Disease. A specialist is more likely to keep abreast of advances in treatment that may be appropriate for your family member.

4. If you are more likely to believe a specialist than your family doctor, a diagnosis by a specialist will reduce the likelihood that you will "shop around" for another doctor, or deny the diagnosis because it makes you unhappy. However, you should seek a second opinion if you think an error has been made, regardless of who made the diagnosis.

Examples of specialists knowledgeable about Alzheimer Disease include neurologists, who treat diseases of the nervous system; behavioural neurologists, who treat neurological diseases that affect behaviour; geriatricians, who specialize in treating older people; and psychogeriatricians–psychiatrists who specialize in mental problems of older people.

The best way to find such a specialist is to ask your family doctor to make a referral. Explain to the doctor that you think your family member may have Alzheimer Disease, and that you would like to be referred to someone who can do a complete assessment and make an accurate diagnosis. You should not feel uncomfortable asking your family doctor to refer you to a specialist. After all, if it were a disease such as cancer that you were concerned about, you would not hesitate to ask for a specialist for that condition. Alzheimer Disease is also a special medical condition.

To help you feel more comfortable about asking your family doctor to make a referral, you might point out to him or her that he will continue to serve as your family doctor for other problems, and that you will be wanting to talk to him and work with him around certain aspects of managing the Alzheimer patient. In fact, it is important that your family doctor feel comfortable in talking with you about the disease, and feel comfortable with the idea of being part of a care team that will also include you, as the primary caregiver, as well as the specialist and other helping and health professionals.

If, despite all this, you still feel uncomfortable asking your family doctor to refer you to another doctor, there are two other ways you can get the names of specialists: phone the medical association in your community and ask them for the names of some doctors who specialize in dealing with Alzheimer Disease; call the nearest chapter of the Alzheimer Society and ask them for the names of some doctors who are knowledgable about Alzheimer Disease.

Neither the medical association nor the Alzheimer Society will recommend specific doctors; instead, they will give you a list of names, and you will have to choose among them. This is why it is preferable to ask your family doctor for a referral.

TYPICAL DIAGNOSTIC TESTS

The exact tests that comprise a comprehensive diagnostic assessment will vary somewhat from facility to facility. However, a typical diagnostic series, which might take place over several different sessions, is likely to include most of the following:

Blood test The purpose of blood tests is to determine whether other medical conditions are causing the problem; whether the patient is suffering from another form of dementia other than Alzheimer Disease; or whether there is a treatable disorder that is aggravating an underlying dementing illness.

Medical history A thorough medical history is probably the single most important element in developing an accurate diagnosis. The history will help determine whether other health problems are causing or contributing to the symptoms. The history will include answers to such questions as how long the condition has persisted, the rate of onset, whether it is cyclical, and similar issues that will assist in the diagnosis.

Social history This history will address questions such as how the patient is functioning, the areas in which the memory loss presents problems, how the patient and the family are coping, and what procedures are being used to help compensate for the memory loss. This portion of the assessment not only contributes to the accuracy of the diagnosis, but also plays an important role in counselling the family on how to cope with the patient's problems.

Psychiatric assessment An assessment by a psychiatrist will contribute to the accurate diagnosis by eliminating psychiatric illnesses such as depression, which mimic Alzheimer Disease. As well, this will also help identify psychiatric problems that may exist in addition to the Alzheimer Disease. Depression, which is common in the elderly in general, is also common among patients in the early stages of Alzheimer Disease when they sense that something is wrong, but do not know what the problem is.

Neuropsychological assessment This battery of tests is used to determine the areas in which the patient's mental functioning has become affected. It will measure attention span, concentration, recent and immediate memory, ability to learn new things, language skills, and motor coordination. Besides contributing to the assessment of the problem, it will provide baseline information against which further changes can be measured in the future.

Mental status assessment The patient will be asked a series of questions about time and place, and about her or his knowledge of major current issues, such as who the Prime Minister is. Like the neurological tests, these questions are intended to identify the areas of brain function that have been affected, and thus will also contribute to the diagnosis.

Other tests A chest x-ray and an EEG (electro-encephalogram) may also be included as part of the diagnostic battery. The chest x-ray will be used to rule out other conditions. In an EEG test, electrodes are attached to the scalp so that the patient's brain waves can be recorded. While this may appear frightening, it is a simple and safe procedure that may provide information on the functioning of the patient's brain.

CAT/CT (Computerized Axial Tomograph) This is a procedure that produces x-rays of cross sections of the brain. These x-rays are then fed into a computer to obtain a picture of the brain tissue. (Conventional x-rays show the bones of the skull, rather than the brain tissue itself.) While there are changes in the appearance of the brain tissue among patients with Alzheimer Disease, the presence of these changes does not necessarily mean the patient has Alzheimer Disease.

When the necessary diagnostic battery has been completed, the doctor will require time to review and interpret the results of the various tests. When this has been completed, he or she will meet with you again to discuss the results, tell you what they mean, and discuss how you should proceed. During these days of waiting, make a list of questions to ask the doctor when you go back to learn the test results.

You will want to know what the diagnosis means, and what the implications are. If the doctor has not given you enough information, don't feel shy about asking questions. If you don't understand the words he uses, ask him to clarify them, or to explain it again in simple English. Review the list of questions you have assembled since your last visit, and make sure all of them have been answered. The doctor may be able to help you begin your search for community resources, and may know how you can contact the Alzheimer Society near your home. Ask him also if you can call him again as you think of additional questions, or whether he can recommend someone else who can help you.

At this time, you may also want to talk to the specialist about his or her role in the ongoing treatment and management of the patient. The questions you might ask about this include:

Will you be the doctor in charge of the patient, or do you only do diagnoses?

When should I bring the patient to see you? Should it be on a regular basis, and if so, when, or should it be when certain milestones occur?

Can I call you in an emergency? Are there others at the centre/clinic I should call instead? Who are they and how do I reach them?

Have you sent a report to my family doctor? Would you be willing to talk to him or her, to help him help me?

THE DIAGNOSIS

As you now know, Alzheimer Disease is difficult to diagnose. Diagnosis is achieved by ruling out other diseases that often appear to be the same as Alzheimer Disease. A completely accurate diagnosis is only achievable through the autopsy of brain tissue at death. However, specialists are reporting an increasingly high percent of accurate diagnoses; some report an accurate diagnosis rate of ninety percent.

To give you some sense of the difficulty of making a diagnosis, and therefore the importance of a comprehensive assessment undertaken by a specialist, note the following list of reversible causes of "apparent dementia"; that is, those conditions that appear to be a dementia but that are really caused by a reversible, treatable condition:

D   drugs/degenerative disorders such as Parkinson's Disease or Multiple Sclerosis
E   emotional illness
M   metabolic and endocrine problems, such as diabetes and thyroid malfunctions
E   eyes/ears/environmental difficulties
N   nutritional and neurological disorders
T   tumours and trauma
I   infections
A   alcohol abuse or withdrawal/anemia

In fact, there are more than sixty other disorders with symptoms similar to those of Alzheimer Disease, and a number of other related disorders that can also cause dementia: multi-infarct dementia, Huntington's Disease, Parkinson's Disease, and Creutzfeld-Jakob Disease. Some of the disorders that initially appear to be Alzheimer Disease, but are not, are reversible or treatable.

A woman was admitted to our Day Program having been diagnosed at the local hospital as having Alzheimer Disease. She had been admitted to the hospital through emergency, when she was found wandering on the street in the middle of the night. When we were doing our intake interview I noticed that her clothes seemed to be quite large for her, and asked her son if she had shown any recent weight loss. He told me she had lost about 25 pounds over the last few months, and when I asked him why, he said his father had died recently and his mother wasn't eating very well—she said it was too much trouble to cook for one. I asked the son why he hadn't told the doctor this at the hospital, and he said the doctor hadn't asked him. Her strange behaviour had occurred because she was malnourished, not because of Alzheimer Disease, and now that we've organized for her to get meals on wheels, she is doing much better.

Depression Depression in the elderly is so often confused with Alzheimer Disease that it has been referred to as pseudodementia. Depressed people will often appear to have a memory loss, though on further investigation, it often turns out that they are unwilling, rather than unable, to answer questions designed to test their memory, and that when motivated or pushed, they are indeed able to perform well on mental assessment scales.

Delirium Delirium is an acute confusional state that usually has a rapid onset and is of short duration. The most common causes are infection and the excess use of drugs, including alcohol, or the too rapid withdrawal of a drug; other medical conditions can also lead to delirium.

OTHER DISEASES

Alzheimer Disease would be enough for your family to deal with, and it would be nice if there were no other medical problems besides this main one. Unfortunately, this is not the case. Not only do people bring into the disease problems or conditions that they had before, but they continue to develop new ones. These new ones are not necessarily a result of the Alzheimer Disease, but may occur because of normal disease processes or normal processes of aging.

Most likely your family doctor will treat your family member for these problems or will refer him to a specialist if the problem warrants it. Basically, the decision to refer an Alzheimer patient to a specialist for any other problem should be made as if the person did not have Alzheimer Disease. However, because stability and continuity are always to be desired in caring for a person with Alzheimer Disease, it may be preferable for the family doctor to treat the Alzheimer patient for problems that might otherwise be referred to a specialist.

As the Alzheimer Disease progresses, your family member will become less able to explain health problems to you or to the doctor. It is therefore important that you observe the patient carefully for signs of other health problems. Look for signs of pain or discomfort in the form of facial expressions or a change in behaviour, such as a limp to avoid putting pressure on a sore foot. Changes in your family member's routine may signal either a change in the Alzheimer Disease or a change in health. Don't make assumptions about the cause without checking with your doctor first.

When my wife became bladder incontinent I was pretty certain it was due to the Alzheimer Disease, but since I wasn't sure I called her doctor. He checked her over and found she had a urinary tract infection.

If it is necessary to ask the Alzheimer patient questions about his or her health, use the same approach you would for other kinds of questions. Avoid open-ended questions that can admit to several answers. Instead, give your family member questions that have a limited range of responses. Don't ask, "What's wrong with you?" Do ask, "Does your foot hurt?"

Use non-verbal communication to supplement your words. For example, if you are not sure whether your family member knows the parts of the body, point to or touch the part you are asking about, and ask if it hurts. You can also observe your family member's facial expression.

FURTHER READING

Melinick, Vijaya and Dubler, Nancy (Eds.). *Alzheimer's Disease: Dilemmas in Clinical Research*. Clifton, New Jersey: Humana Press, 1985.

Reisberg, Barry. *A Guide to Alzheimer's Disease: For Families, Spouses and Friends*. New York: Free Press, 1984.

5

COMMUNITY RESOURCES:
USING THE SYSTEM

❦

ach person on the team caring for the person with Alzheimer
Disease needs the help of the other team members: the
primary caregiver, the relatives, friends, neighbours and
professionals. Therefore the community resources are essential.

Living with Alzheimer Disease means managing a long, difficult, and devastating illness. You have the right to the best and most
appropriate help available in your community. And it's yours if you
know how to use it. You also have the right to ensure that you do not
become a "patient" yourself.

In this chapter "using the system" means choosing the services
of selected professionals, finding community programs and services, utilizing family support groups, and using the neighbourhood
to your advantage.

You will learn what networking means and how you can use it
to tap into the system of services available in your community. You
will find out how to obtain needed respite so that your physical and
emotional strengths remain intact.

BUILDING A SUPPORT SYSTEM:
NETWORKING

When my husband was first diagnosed with Alzheimer Disease, I
was able to manage without any help. He came shopping and
on errands with me, and was able to remain at home alone on
occasion without any problems.

The "slippers incident" changed all that. I returned from the
bank one wintry day to find that my husband had left the house to

go for a walk wearing his slippers, and no coat. My next door neighbour spotted him, and took him into her house until I returned home.

I knew I could no longer leave him alone. Over tea with the neighbour who found him, I learned that her cousin's wife, whose husband had Alzheimer Disease, was using the services of a community respite program. She promised to give me her cousin's phone number so I could find out about the program. As we talked further, my neighbour mentioned that she would not mind spending one morning a week with my husband so that I could get out.

Although I was retired and able to stay home with my wife who had Alzheimer Disease, I had never been very good in the kitchen. The stress of having to make meals as well as look after my wife was getting to me. Although my daughter-in-law had offered to cook some meals for me, I felt that she was too busy and that this would be an imposition. A pamphlet I had received from the local Alzheimer chapter mentioned a number to call for a service that would deliver daily hot meals to my home. My daughter-in-law made the call for me. Those hot meals saved my life.

In my family physician's office, I saw a flyer advertising a lecture sponsored by the Public Health Department on caring for a relative with Alzheimer Disease. Although I couldn't arrange to attend the lecture, I called the Public Health Department for more information. The end result was a home visit. The nurse who came gave me practical suggestions about my daily routine at home, and gave me the number of a day program that had just been started in my neighbourhood.

Building your support system has to do with finding and using resources that will help you be a more effective caregiver, and to feel less alone with your problem. The way to build yourself a support system is through "networking." Start by making a list of people who can act as initial resources for you in your community such as the public health nurse, your neighbours, your local Alzheimer chapter. After you have made your list, call the people or organizations. These calls will give you further leads to follow up, and this is how your support system or network is built.

You may feel distressed, tired, and confused. Perhaps you feel that you do not need the added burden of making telephone calls or writing letters. If starting your network seems overwhelming, break tasks down into smaller steps that can be accomplished one at a time. Start with one phone call a day and follow up leads from there. This is an opportunity to ask for help from the neighbour who has said "If there is anything I can do. . . ."

HOW TO START

Use this list of places and people in your community as a beginning and add to it as you make more contacts.

1. The public health nurse in your area
2. Your local Alzheimer chapter
3. The social work department in the hospital closest to you
4. Victorian Order of Nurses office in your area
5. Your local government representative
6. The seniors bureau, office for seniors, or provincial department responsible for services for seniors in your community
7. Your local community information or referral centre
8. Your clergyman
9. Your family physician or the nurse in your physician's office
10. The doctor or clinic where the Alzheimer patient was initially assessed

TELEPHONE TIPS

If the person you start with cannot help, make sure that you ask for the name and phone number of someone else who may have the information you are looking for. Don't become discouraged if one call leads to several others. Networking is a process. It takes time and patience, but making the calls will help you feel more in control.

Always get the name of the person you are speaking to, and use that name when you are making follow-up calls. For example:

"Hello. My name is Mr. Brown. I was given your name by Mrs. Rose in the Greenville Area Public Health Department. My wife has Alzheimer Disease, and I understand you have information about a program that provides care in the home."

Try to be specific about what you are looking for, but be prepared at the same time to receive new information.

"Yes, Mr. Brown. I'm not the one to speak to about care in the home, but we do have a small day program for persons with Alzheimer Disease. Tell me about your wife.''

Don't be afraid to call your referral source back, and report that the person they told you to call did not have the information you require. Ask for further help.

COMMUNITY SERVICES

Once you know the people to call, and how to call them, you will have taken the first step in identifying the kinds of services that might be available in your community. The range of services varies from province to province, and even from municipality to municipality. You will find a reference at the end of this chapter to service and resource guides for each province.

PRACTICAL HELP

Not only is it important to become aware of what community resources are available and how to access them, but it is essential to know when to choose one specific service or program over another, and when one resource option will benefit the family and the person with Alzheimer Disease more than others. For example, in some cases it might be more helpful to have home respite-care than to send the person with Alzheimer Disease to a day program, assuming that both services are available. There are many factors and variables to be considered, and these will be discussed in appropriate sections of this chapter. A list of some of the services you can look for follows.

1. *Meals* "Meals on Wheels" is a community service that brings meals into your home on a regular basis. This program can relieve you of having to provide a nourishing hot meal every day while you are caring for an Alzheimer patient. You may also be able to obtain the services of a homemaker who can help prepare meals for the family on a regular basis.

   There are also programs that can take the Alzheimer patient to a meal service in the community (Wheels to Meals or Diner Club). This kind of program can offer a social experience as well as a balanced meal.

   If your family member needs close supervision because of wandering and/or difficult behaviour, the "wheels to meals" option may not be appropriate. You should check to see if the number of staff and volunteers are adequate to care appropriately for the person.

2. *Homemaker Services* Services of a homemaker may be available to prepare meals, shop, do laundry, provide light housekeeping or heavy cleaning, and provide personal care services such as dressing. Taking advantage of this kind of service will help you conserve energy, and have more time for the patient and for yourself. In the earlier stages you may need a homemaker only once a week for light housekeeping duties. Later, when it is harder to leave your family member alone, you might need to increase the number of days a homemaker comes, and the tasks that you assign.

3. *Health Services* Your community may offer visiting nursing programs that send nurses to your home on a regular basis. There are also specialty health services such as occupational therapists and podiatrists that visit seniors in their homes. Some medical clinics provide home visits.

4. *Home Maintenance* There may be a service in your area that provides volunteers to help with small jobs around the house such as carpentry and repairs.

5. *Emergency Services* Some communities offer emergency medical services to the home, as well as crisis help lines and mobile crisis services. Your Alzheimer chapter or local police department may know of any specialized emergency programs in your community.

6. *Transportation* Find out if there is special transportation available in your community for the elderly and the disabled, and if people with Alzheimer Disease are eligible for this service.

7. *Respite-Care Services* Respite-care is periodic, short-term care for the purpose of providing relief for the family caregiver who is caring for a relative at home. Care should be at a level and location appropriate to individual needs.

RESPITE IN YOUR HOME

Nobody will ever look after your sick relative as well as you do, but you still need relief. In-home respite-care is an important source of relief. There are ways to ensure that the respite experience is as satisfying and safe as possible for the person with Alzheimer Disease, the family caregiver, and the respite-worker. Once you have identified some options, use the following questions to get the information you need (these will apply to a commercial as well as a non-profit agency).

1. Does the agency conduct personal interviews to determine the suitability of a person as a respite-worker helping people who have Alzheimer Disease?

2. Does the agency check references before hiring staff?

3. Are respite-workers in the agency bonded or bondable?

4. What specific training and orientation are respite-workers given before they are placed in homes?

5. Does the supervisor conduct an in-home visit to become acquainted with the home environment and meet the caregiver and the person with Alzheimer Disease?

6. Is a functional assessment done, preferably in the home, or by an in-depth telephone conversation? This assessment will ascertain what level of ability your family member has in performing activities such as eating, dressing, bathing, communicating, and toileting. This assessment will help the agency to have a better understanding of your family member's needs.

7. Is the agency able to offer a consistent person who will be able to have a regular arrangement for specific days of the week? It is extremely important that the worker and the arrangement be consistent so that the Alzheimer patient can become used to the same person and form a relationship with her or him. A consistent schedule will also be helpful to both you and the patient.

8. Is staff supervision provided by the agency?

9. Will the respite-worker be trained and undertake to carry out personal care tasks such as assistance in the washroom, assistance with transferring, help with dressing, grooming, eating, and similar daily activities?

10. Is there some provision for back-up? What happens if you are late getting back, or if you need a respite-worker evenings, nights and weekends?

11. Is there a cancellation fee? How much notice of cancellation is required?

12. Does the agency check to see if you were pleased with the respite-worker and if all went well?

The first time you use the services of a respite-worker you will likely feel nervous. It will help if you are prepared to spend at least thirty minutes talking to the respite-worker before you go out. During this time you could show him or her around the house or apartment and introduce the Alzheimer patient. You will make the respite-worker's task easier if you include the following information in an orientation.

1. A personal history: What are some important biographical details that will help the respite-worker to have a rounded picture of the person with Alzheimer Disease?

2. Give an explanation of what tasks the Alzheimer patient is able to perform independently and for what the person needs help.

3. Leave a written list of what medication the Alzheimer patient takes and what medication may be needed during the time the respite-worker is present.

4. Mention any idiosyncratic behaviour, such as body language, that will help the worker to communicate effectively. This may take some thought since you probably have become used to some expressions or traits and automatically respond to them.

5. If it is possible, you may want to leave a phone number where you can be reached. Also leave a list of essential people such as physicians, relatives and neighbours, and of course, emergency numbers.

If you are not pleased with the respite service you have tried, investigate other commercial and non-profit agencies. Do not assume that if you pay more to a commercial agency, you will get better service, or that a large organization can necessarily provide more than a small one. Use the guidelines above to help choose a service that will suit your needs.

If you have any reservations about the respite-worker the agency sends, a good agency will be happy to discuss them with you. But be reasonable. Nobody will ever be as good a caregiver or know your relative as well as you do. However, if the respite-worker is impatient, not willing or able to communicate very well, or shows little interest in the ill person, it is reasonable to ask for another worker or to try another service.

It is your responsibility to try to be back on time when you go out since the respite-worker may be expected by another family. The first time you use a respite-worker, you might want to stay out a short time so that you have time to talk to the worker and to be assured that your relative is all right. If you are late, you may be asked to pay extra, since the agency may pay the worker on an hourly basis. It is best to discuss this if you think there is a possibility that you will be late.

THE "SET-UP"

It is your responsibility to tell the respite-worker about difficulties that could occur while you are out and how you usually deal with these kind of situations. You might feel threatened by the idea of leaving your relative in someone else's care. You might not like being replaced in your caregiver role. Both situations could be scary for you. Try to avoid the "set-up": not sharing all the information a caregiver needs and thus showing that you are the only one who can look after your relative.

If you feel that it will make the transition easier, you may want to stay home during the worker's first visit to allow you to have some private time at home, and then go out on the second visit.

> I very carefully explained to my husband that I was going to the bank and to the shopping mall and that Helen (the respite-worker we were trying for the first time) would be staying with him. He smiled and seemed fine when I left. However, when I returned a few hours later, I found my husband in a state of panic. He was pacing back and forth at the front door waiting for me to return. I felt terrible.

The first time you leave your relative with a respite-worker is very difficult, but as both of you become accustomed to it, the experience will become easier. Even with the most conscientious preparation, expect that the Alzheimer patient may be agitated or upset the first time respite is provided. Your relative is used to your being there for him or her all the time; you will be missed. A good respite-worker who is adquately trained should be able to handle any difficulties. Even though it is very difficult, keep your appointment to go out.

Keep trying. In the best situations the worker and the patient will become good friends. Let the agency know if the respite experience went well and give positive feedback to the worker as well. Remember that you need the time away to look after yourself.

This will help to prevent two patients and will give you some perspective as a caregiver and as a person.

INSTITUTIONAL RESPITE

Most in-home respite programs provide care for only a few hours; the maximum may be twenty-four hours. If you need respite for longer than that, you may be able to obtain institutional respite-care through a long-term care facility such as a chronic hospital, a nursing home, or a home for the aged.

You might want to use this service if you are planning a vacation; if you feel you need an extended break from caregiving; or if you know that you will be unable to provide care because of something like elective surgery. (In Chapter 11, "Special Problems," you will find suggestions on what to do when an emergency makes you unable to continue to be an Alzheimer patient's caregiver.)

Each facility has its own policies about providing institutional respite-care. You should contact them to find out their policy as soon as you begin to think about using the service, so that you don't make plans based on incorrect assumptions.

There are a number of things you need to think about before deciding to use an institutional respite service.

1. The Alzheimer patient may become disoriented away from home. New routines and people are difficult to cope with, and may be upsetting. A patient may also have difficulty readjusting to the home routine.

2. You may feel tense and guilty about leaving your relative in the care of strangers, even though they are trained professionals. This may undermine the purpose of the respite in the first place.

3. Some caregivers have been surprised to find that it was hard to return to a routine of caregiving after they experienced some tension release for a period of time. They hadn't realized how much strain they were under until they were relieved.

Clearly this is a situation where you must consider the trade-offs before making a decision. Whatever you decide, be aware that you will have to take your family member home when the respite period contracted for is over. Someone else in the community is probably booked into the bed your family member has been using. Besides, respite-care should never be considered a back door to institutionalization.

DAY PROGRAMS

Specialized day programs for Alzheimer patients have been initiated in several centres across Canada. In fact, the numbers are growing so rapidly that any list we included in this book would be quickly out of date.

Check with the local Alzheimer Society chapter in your area for information about a day program for Alzheimer patients in your community. In most cases, day programs for the non-impaired elderly will not be able to accommodate an Alzheimer patient since programming is geared to people who can participate in groups, and can easily find their way around the facility. Use this list to assess an Alzheimer day program.

1. Is the staffing adequate? Consider both professional and volunteer staff. Look for a staff-to-client ratio of 1:3 to 1:5.

2. Is this a secure facility that can protect an Alzheimer patient's safety if he or she wanders?

3. Is the facility accessible to wheelchairs?

4. Is there a structured routine to the day with flexibility for individual needs?

5. Is transportation provided? If you are not going to accompany the patient, is there provision for someone to receive and bring home the person right to the door? Some programs may expect you to drive the patient there and back. You should assess the hours of the program and the suitability of this arrangement for your lifestyle and for your relative.

6. Are nutritious meals and snacks provided? Is there provision for special diets?

You need to think about how often your family member should go to a day program. Think about what will work for you both. More than once a week will help the person with Alzheimer Disease to become accustomed to the routine. On the other hand, four times a week may be too much, and cause fatigue and disorientation. Expect some tiredness from the stress of new stimuli, and experiment with the number of days, and the number of hours each day.

There may need to be trade-offs between the amount of time you need for respite during the week, and the amount of time the Alzheimer patient can go to a day program without becoming fatigued.

Do not be discouraged if the Alzheimer patient has difficulty adapting to the program. Work with staff to help the person feel comfortable, and try different approaches before deciding whether or not to use the program.

Be open with staff, and alert them to any aspects of care they need to know about to provide a high quality service. Do not set yourself up for failure by not sharing your expertise with them. Be a partner-in-caring.

THE ALZHEIMER SOCIETY

Another specialized source of help is the Alzheimer Society of Canada, founded in 1980 to provide support to families, promote research into the cause and cure of Alzheimer Disease, and inform and educate the community. There are about seventy-five chapters across Canada covering every province; if there is a chapter in your community you will find a listing in the telephone directory. An updated national list of Alzheimer chapters with contact names, addresses, and phone numbers is provided for you in the Appendix.

If you have difficulty locating the chapter or contact person in your area, or if you need any information about chapters in your surrounding area, you can call the national office of the Alzheimer Society of Canada. Resource material at the national office can inform you about the disease and how to cope, as well as provide guidelines about how to start a chapter in your area, if there isn't one.

Local chapters hold regular meetings and distribute resource material, including a regular newsletter for members. They also keep track of events and services in their area, and often sponsor or organize family support groups for relatives of people who have Alzheimer Disease.

Alzheimer chapters are always looking for people to volunteer on committees; to help with special program or fund-raising projects; or to serve as a member of the Board of Directors. Some people find that getting involved at the local, provincial, or national level helps to "make sense" of a painful life situation in a meaningful way.

Although some of my friends went to family support groups, I was always uncomfortable with this. However, serving on the Board of Directors of my chapter and later provincially, helped me a lot. I was able to do something constructive about Alzheimer Disease and felt satisfied with what I could accomplish.

Consider your energy and stress level before making a volunteer commitment. You may be overwhelmed with the changes occurring in your life and although you are able to benefit from attending chapter functions, you may lack energy to be a regular volunteer. In fact, some people become more involved after they are no longer providing direct care to a family member.

FAMILY SUPPORT GROUPS

Family support groups are mutual support groups in which family caregivers can meet with each other to share experiences and feelings, exchange practical information, and solve problems. Instead of the lecture format of an educational meeting, members are encouraged to discuss their own situations and to learn from each other. Some of these groups are organized directly by the Alzheimer Society, while others are sponsored by long-term-care facilities, hospitals, or community-based agencies.

The Alzheimer Society in your area should have a list of available groups, together with the name of a contact person and information about when and where the groups meet. Groups are usually designed to accommodate members who are available either during the daytime or in the evenings.

People who come to the group are not special kinds of people. They are not necessarily people who have attended groups before, nor are they especially outgoing. The support group is for those who are coping with a very difficult situation—living with a family member who has Alzheimer Disease. In a support group you discover that you are not alone.

Mrs. A We came back from shopping and I didn't know whether to laugh or cry. My husband unloaded the groceries and put them in the garbage.

Mr. B I know just how you felt. My wife tried to help me in the kitchen and threw out half our dinner.

Mrs. A It's hard because you want to let them help, and yet it's so much easier and faster to do it yourself.

Mrs. C Not only that. I get impatient and then I feel terrible when I lose my temper.

Mr. B That's the worst part. Getting angry and then feeling guilty.

Mrs. A I'm so glad to hear you say that. I thought I was the only one who had these guilty feelings.

In a support group you also find out about tips and techniques that other families have used in daily situations.

Mrs. P	My husband forgets that he's eaten and he's gaining weight from nibbling snack food.
Mrs. N	I found it helpful to offer my husband some celery or carrot sticks. That way he won't gain weight, and we avoid a painful argument.
Mr. M	I'll try that next time and see if it works for me.

Some support groups have a professional facilitator available to answer questions and suggest topics of relevance for the group; in these groups the facilitator and the group members usually agree on a set number of sessions. The facilitator may be a social worker, a trained group leader, a counsellor, or a lay person who has participated in groups and has been trained to lead groups. Often the group members exchange phone numbers and keep in contact with each other after the formal sessions have ended.

Other groups are on-going and are run by members. Members come every week and discuss their experiences and feelings without the assistance of a professional facilitator. Sometimes when the professionally led group is finished, the group continues on its own.

It sounds good but it makes me anxious.

If you feel threatened by the idea of a support group, or are not sure if this is a comfortable way for you to receive and give help, there are several things you can do to test it out.

Talk about your concerns to the person in the local Alzheimer chapter or long-term-care facility responsible for organizing the support groups. Ask for a personal interview to discuss the support groups.

Talk to someone already in a group or someone who has been in a group (the chapter should be able to get permission from members to give out names and phone numbers for this purpose) and ask them whatever questions you have about the experience. If the group has a professional or lay facilitator, make an appointment to meet with him or her and discuss your questions about attending a family support group.

Ask a friend or relative to attend with you. This will provide support for you in the group, and may provide you with an informed helper outside of group sessions. Your informed helper could remind you of experiences you want to bring to the next group session, assist you to use new techniques or tips you learn from other group members, and provide moral and social support.

Many family members want to attend a support group but worry about who will look after the Alzheimer patient, especially if the groups are held in the evening. Later in this chapter you will find information on the informal network as a source of respite help for this kind of occasion. Attending a group is a time-limited event and it may be possible to call upon a neighbour, close friend, or relative.

What could be even more difficult to deal with is your worry about what is happening at home while you are in the group: what if my husband has an accident with the stove, or wanders away from the person looking after him, or gets into a panic when I have been gone for awhile? Expressing the stress you are feeling while in the group may help to relieve the tension, and will permit others to discuss their feelings about their own situations.

STARTING A SUPPORT GROUP

If you think you would benefit from a family support group and have not been able to find one in your community, you may be interested in helping to start one in conjunction with other care-givers and professionals in your area. The national office has a handbook that offers advice. If you feel too anxious to be the one to do it, show it to someone in your community who may have the appropriate resources.

Here are some suggestions.

1. Don't re-invent the wheel. Speak to others who have started a group for family caregivers and obtain sample materials such as flyers and press releases they have used.

2. Form a core group or steering committee to prevent yourself from burning out. If you take on the job of starting a group without help from others, you may find that it is too much for you to handle, along with your caregiving tasks. Sharing the activities with a small group of other caregivers will make the job easier, and will keep your enthusiasm and energies intact.

3. Find a suitable time and meeting place that is available and appropriate for you, such as a community centre, social service centre, hospital, or library. If you are more comfortable in informal surroundings, investigate the possibility of meeting in caregivers' homes on a rotating basis.

4. Consider the best way to reach potential members. Use public health nurses, physicians, flyers, free announcements in newspapers, and public service announcements on TV and radio to get your message out.

5. It's natural to have ups and downs in attendance and enthusiasm. Some members of the group will have to stay home at times because of caregiving responsibilities. Some people will gain insight from the group, and then feel that they no longer need to come. Some members may come only when they are experiencing a crisis.

YOUR PERSONAL SUPPORT SYSTEM

Though your community services are important, developing a personal support system is equally important.

People often forget about or are hesitant to call on family members, neighbours, and friends. Informal helpers can be significant sources of emotional support and strength and can provide "normalcy" time for caregivers whose days are lacking in diversion and social interchange.

The services outlined in this chapter are only available at set times and for limited periods during the week. Your caregiving routine doesn't stop on weekends and evenings. Informal helpers can fill in the gap and give you a needed break when professional services are not available. Another way to find help for the evenings is to contact agencies who provide respite-care during the day.

To start your personal network, make a list of everyone who you might ask for some kind of help.

1. Your closest family members, such as children and grandchildren

2. More distant, but "close" relatives, such as cousins, aunts and uncles

3. Friends you see regularly

4. Friends you see less often

5. Neighbours you know well and who know your family member

6. Fellow members of a recreational club, organization, or association that you belong to, whether it is an organized social club or informal card group

7. Members of your church or synagogue

8. Local shopkeepers and professionals such as bank tellers who know you and your family member

9. People in your work setting

> My husband was a minister. Although he could no longer carry on after he was diagnosed with Alzheimer Disease, we remained members of the same church and attended services whenever possible. My husband still enjoyed the singing, but was becoming more and more restless and agitated during the service. I thought we would soon have to stop coming to church together, an activity that meant a lot to both of us.
>
> One Sunday a member of the congregation we knew quite well who had noticed the restlessness offered to help. She suggested that we sit near her at the back. When my husband started to get restless, she took him out for a walk so that I could enjoy the rest of the service.
>
> When this was no longer possible, she organized a small team of church volunteers to alternate staying with my husband on Sunday mornings so I could still attend services.
>
> I would never have thought of asking for assistance from people in the congregation, yet, once they offered it was easy to let them help.

Remember that people cannot read your mind. If you need help you have to ask for it. In most cases people will be willing to lend a hand if they know that you need help, and if they are given a specific task.

Think about what kinds of things you most need help with. For example, you may have been intending to call someone to find out how to arrange for a homemaker service in your community. Every time you get out the phone number, something interferes and then you put it off for another day. This is something you can ask someone to do for you.

Neighbours can help by spending time at home with the Alzheimer patient to allow you to have relief out of the house for banking, shopping, appointments, or recreation; or by doing some shopping, banking or other errands in the neighbourhood. Also, an informed and empathetic neighbour can be an important community partner who can take on the role of explaining the patient's bizarre behaviour to others in the community and generally watching out for him or her.

You need support from those around you. The people in your personal network know other people. This increases your chances of gaining knowledge and support in your community.

My employer was very sympathetic when I finally told him about my wife. A couple of days later, he called me to say that he had mentioned Alzheimer Disease to the person in charge of the Employee Assistance Program in my company. She sent me a list of agencies that send workers into the home, and also told me about a spouse's support group.

If you inform local shopkeepers about your family member's condition, they will be able to understand unusual behaviour and will be better able to handle problems that arise.

My husband enjoyed helping me by walking to the variety store a few blocks from our house and shopping for small items like a loaf of bread or some milk. It made him feel useful and in touch with the neighbourhood. I would write the items down on a piece of paper and he would give this to the owner—a man we have known for many years who was aware that my husband had Alzheimer Disease.

Often my husband would forget to pay the owner, even though I had checked to make sure there was money in his wallet. We solved this problem by working out a credit system. The storeowner kept track of what we owed, and I went in and paid the whole amount once a month. This allowed my husband to retain his dignity and feel useful.

Remember that tasks that seemed small before you became a caregiver can now seem overwhelming. You may feel silly about asking a friend to help you balance the books, or write thank you letters, or contact the Alzheimer Society, but this can make a big difference in an already overloaded day.

A small group of consistent friends may be able to stay with your family member when you go out. Even if you have a profession-al respite-worker, there will be times when you need to supplement this service with friends. Remember that the "set-up" alert that applied to respite-workers applies to friends as well. Be sure to tell them what they need to know, so that they can do a good job while you are out. Helpers need to know the rules of the game.

For example, if you know that the Alzheimer patient finds it relaxing to play with a deck of cards, inform your friend who is relieving you and leave the cards in easy reach. If you suspect that the patient might ask for lunch even though the meal is over, have vegetable sticks available in the kitchen and tell your friend to offer these to your family member. Alert your informal helper if your family member wanders, and leave a list of emergency numbers just as you would for a respite-worker.

You may need to consider your comfort level with letting friends stay with your relative. You will be letting them into a very private part of your life. The friends you select should be accepting and tolerant, as well as trustworthy and responsible. If you are not sure that a friend can handle the job, or if you will feel too exposed, ask them to help in other ways.

Consider also that if a respite-worker stays with your family member, and something goes wrong, you have the option of complaining to the agency. If it is a friend or neighbour, you have to consider how you will handle it. Try to avoid hurt feelings, but remember that you always have to think about the safety and care of the ill person first.

Tell your friends who help you that you appreciate their help, but do not feel obligated to continually repay them. Small ways of showing your appreciation can be very effective. A card expressing your thanks, or flowers once in a while, will do the trick. Remember that informal helpers are choosing to give you a break. You are letting them feel good about themselves, by giving them a chance to help. This is an important part of the interaction.

Building your community and personal network will help you feel in control, and will maximize both your ability to care for your relative, and your own quality of life.

PRODUCTS TO MAKE
CAREGIVING EASIER

Numerous products have been developed for people who are ill and need assistance with daily activities such as eating, bathing, dressing, toileting and even leisure activities. These products are usually sold through specialty stores, which usually have catalogues that you can order. Look in the Yellow Pages of the phone book under Hospital Equipment and Supplies to get the name of a store in your community.

If your community is too small to have a store like this, use your network to find the nearest place where you can buy these products. The purchasing agent at the nearest hospital may be able to help you. You could also try asking someone at the Public Health

Department, or an occupational therapist. If all else fails, contact
the hospital or clinic where the Alzheimer patient's diagnosis was
made and ask to see a catalogue.

Your first step should be to look through the catalogue to find
the range of products that are available. Once you have identified
the type of product you need, you should consult with a knowledgeable professional (an occupational therapist, a nurse, or a salesper-
son in the shop) about whether the product will really meet your
needs, and which of the several alternatives is best for the patient.

If the product you are buying is large or if it must fit with
something else in your home (will the bath seat fit into your bath
tub), then you would probably find an in-home assessment useful.
This would also be appropriate for small items if you are unable to
take the patient to the store with you. On the other hand, if you want
to buy a special fork and plate to make eating easier for the patient,
perhaps the person can go to the store with you.

Sometimes a problem cannot be solved with a product, or you
may not be sure which product to buy. There are people–occupational therapists, specially trained nurses–who can come to your
home and help you with your caregiving problems. They will work
with you to determine whether special equipment will help with
the problem, or whether you need to change the way you deal with a
particular caregiving task. If you need to change your behaviour,
they will help you identify new approaches or teach you new
skills.

In some provinces, the provincial government will pay for
these consultations and for at least some of the aids. Use your
network to find out what the guidelines are in your province.

FURTHER READING

"Alzheimer Support Groups: Leadership Training Guide." A
    pamphlet distributed by The Alzheimer Society of Canada,
    Toronto.
Mace, Nancy. "Self Help for the Family," in Kelly, William (Ed.)
    *Alzheimer's Disease and Related Disorders: Research and
    Management.* Springfield, Illinois: C.C. Thomas, 1984.
Government service guide books (federal and provincial); Seniors
    Secretariat Offices (see listings in Appendix); Alzheimer
    Chapters (see listings in Appendix).

6
LEGAL HELP

❦

As a caregiver, there are important legal and financial decisions that you must make. Dementia will affect the ability of an Alzheimer patient to make judgments, understand choices, and to handle money and legal matters. Therefore it is best to take action in the early stages of the illness to ensure that these matters are under control.

This chapter will prepare you for your visit to the lawyer by explaining the meaning of legal terms and the reason why certain actions on your part will be needed. You will also find suggestions for choosing a lawyer, and information on what might be expected of you as a caregiver. Information on money is also included: what financial decisions you will need to consider, and how to deal with them.

Use this chapter as a planning guide, not as a replacement for consultation with your lawyer. You will find suggestions for using a network approach: exploring what resources are available, how to find them, and how to use them.

DEFINING POWER OF ATTORNEY

A power of attorney is a legal document authorizing one person to act as the attorney or agent of another, under whatever conditions or restrictions are specified. It can be as broad or specific as the person granting the power of attorney requests. Obtaining a power of attorney will ensure that when an Alzheimer patient can no longer make appropriate financial decisions, there is a mechanism in place for someone to sign legal documents and handle legal and financial matters.

> My husband seemed to be carrying on quite normally for several months after the diagnosis of Alzheimer Disease was confirmed. One day I was cleaning the den and found a pile of unpaid bills and second notices for payment neatly stacked under the desk blotter. I became anxious and realized that he was not going to be able to carry on with this responsibility much longer. I discussed my concern with my children and we decided that I should consult our family lawyer. I had already spoken to my husband about the disease and so it wasn't too hard to explain why a visit to the lawyer was necessary.

If you are the person with an appropriately worded power of attorney, you will have the authority to act on behalf of the Alzheimer patient in all legal and financial matters such as signing cheques, selling the house, renewing a mortgage, or entering into a legal contract on his or her behalf.

SEEKING LEGAL ADVICE

WHEN SHOULD I GO TO A LAWYER?

The person who is granting the power of attorney to another person must be legally competent to manage his or her affairs at the time the power of attorney is granted. It is important that power of attorney be arranged while your family member with Alzheimer Disease is aware and can actively participate in the process.

You may be hesitant to initiate discussion with the Alzheimer patient about obtaining power of attorney for yourself or another family member. You may feel guilty about taking away from the person yet another symbol of independence too early. Remember that intellectual ability will decline with Alzheimer Disease, and in the later stages of the disease there will be no opportunity to discuss these things with him or her, or to obtain power of attorney. Involving the person in the decision from the beginning will help to alleviate feelings of guilt on your part. If you need help with this, ask a relative or friend to talk to your ill family member with you.

You might be worried about what other relatives may think. You might be afraid that they will criticize you for rushing to take legal control while the Alzheimer patient stills looks healthy and normal. If this is bothering you, ask another person who knows the facts to speak for you and to explain what you are doing and why.

Perhaps a family meeting will be helpful so that you can share your concern with others and get some advice.

You may not understand what is involved in the process of obtaining power of attorney and it may seem too complicated for you to handle at this time. If this is the case, take the process one step at a time, but do not put off going to a lawyer. Ask a friend or family member to go with you, or to do some initial research for you.

You may be wondering if it is possible to complete the process for obtaining power of attorney without the assistance of a lawyer. We do not recommend this option. If application for a power of attorney is done at home with a home-made form, there are several risks involved.

First of all, the witness may not be considered proper and independent. For example, if the witness is named as the attorney, this is not acceptable. Secondly, it could be claimed later that the person with Alzheimer Disease may have been under duress, or that he or she did not understand what was signed.

If a lawyer prepares the power of attorney, and witnesses it, he or she will be able to testify if the power of attorney is ever challenged in court. Your lawyer can testify that he met with the person with Alzheimer Disease, that the person understood the power of attorney document, and that the person with Alzheimer Disease was not under any undue pressure to the best of his knowledge and belief. Independent corroboration from a lawyer could be very important if a power of attorney is challenged in court.

WHICH LAWYER SHOULD I CHOOSE?

In most cases your family lawyer should be able to serve you without any need for a specialist lawyer. You should, however, make sure that the lawyer you consult understands the situation and is knowledgeable about dementia and its legal implications. If you do not have a family lawyer, or for any reason are not comfortable with your present lawyer you have these options.

1. Check with your local Alzheimer chapter to see if there is a lawyer on their Board of Directors or a lawyer who is closely associated with them.

2. Find out if members of your family support group or other Alzheimer chapter members have been using a lawyer whom

they trust and who understands the legal issues that accompany dementia.

3. Ask relatives and friends for a referral to a lawyer they have used and with whom they feel confident.

4. Check with the Law Society in your province for referrals to lawyers in your community.

Remember that, just as when you choose a physician or a therapist, you have a right to feel comfortable and assured with a lawyer. In most cases, obtaining a power of attorney is not a complicated or expensive process. Find out early what the lawyer's fees are, and what you can expect for this fee. Find out what the lawyer expects of you. Don't be afraid to ask questions even if they seem obvious.

Remember that you are obligated to inform your lawyer that your family member has Alzheimer Disease. If you don't reveal this to your lawyer, the power of attorney may be contested at a later date.

THE LEGAL PROCESSES

WHO SHOULD HAVE POWER OF ATTORNEY?

The person who is given power of attorney should be financially responsible and totally trustworthy. The person with Alzheimer Disease must concur about the choice of the person who is granted power of attorney, and must be aware of what is happening.

We have stressed that the power of attorney is granted when the person with Alzheimer Disease is aware and mentally competent. You might be worried that the power of attorney won't last, once the person with Alzheimer Disease is no longer considered mentally competent. The answer to this varies from province to province. Some provinces allow a power of attorney to continue under certain specified conditions even after the person with Alzheimer Disease is no longer able to understand. You should consult with your lawyer. The power of attorney may remain valid in some provinces if it specifically provides for this in the event of subsequent legal incapacity.

ALTERNATE OR BACK-UP ATTORNEYS

If you are the spouse of someone with Alzheimer Disease, and you are the one to be named as Power of Attorney, it is wise for the person with Alzheimer Disease to designate another person or other people as alternates. This is in case you should die, be unwilling, or be unable for some other reason to carry on as the person with Power of Attorney. For example, the document could name one or more of your children as alternate attorneys to take your place. Otherwise there would be nobody left to exercise the authority of the Power of Attorney, and it would become null and void.

SIBLING RIVALRY–A COMPLICATION

In families where the children do not get along, the children who are not named as attorneys may become upset or jealous about this. It has happened that children not named as attorneys have filed suit to have the power of attorney set aside, claiming that the Alzheimer patient did not know what he was doing at the time. One way to increase the chance that the power of attorney will be upheld by a court is to be sure it is drafted and witnessed by a lawyer. The kind of form you can buy in a stationery store with a neighbour as a witness may not be upheld because the witness may lack credibility.

Sibling rivalry is of course to be avoided if at all possible. The key here is co-operation. There is nothing to be gained by getting into legal disputes, and it can be a costly and stressful matter. Try to consult with all interested children, and attempt to bring in all parties who feel that they should be involved, to avoid this kind of occurrence.

If children are living out of town, the limits of geography usually preclude naming them as alternate attorneys. It would be difficult for them to assume daily responsibilities from a distance. However, if they feel very strongly about being named as one of the attorneys, it might be a good idea to comply, to avoid an ugly dispute.

If there is no responsible person who can assume alternate power of attorney, or if there is a problem with the children, a trust company can be given power of attorney. Usually a trust company will handle this only if there is significant family income and enough assets to justify their involvement. It is preferable to have a trust company as opposed to an individual lawyer or accountant appointed as back-up power of attorney. Trust companies are bonded to ensure against dishonesty or fraud. There is no such assurance if an individual lawyer or accountant is appointed as power of attorney.

GUARDIANSHIP OR COMMITTEESHIP

A committee (the emphasis is on the last syllable) or guardian (the term varies with the jurisdiction) is a person or corporation appointed by a judge to manage assets or exercise certain personal rights on behalf of a person incapable of managing his or her own affairs. This could include management of financial assets as well as authority over personal rights such as the right to give consent to medical treatment.

If there is no power of attorney or if there are problems with the power of attorney that make it impossible to continue with it, then a committeeship is the usual alternative.

If no one applies to the courts for committeeship, in some cases the *Public Trustee* (or equivalent, depending on the province) may by law become the committee or guardian under the requirements of the Mental Health Act of the province. Other names you might come across for this position are *Estate Administrator* and *Curateur Publique*. The Public Trustee is only responsible for financial affairs, but in this capacity can exercise all rights over property, including the right to prosecute or defend court actions in the name of the mentally incompetent person. The Public Trustee can be granted control of the estate of a person with Alzheimer Disease if there is reason to believe that an attorney is mismanaging an estate.

In other cases, an application is made to a judge for an order stating that the person with Alzheimer Disease is not able to handle his or her financial affairs, and naming a private individual or trust company as committee. A plan is described by which the committee is to manage the patient's affairs. The committee is then legally obligated to stay within the provisions of that plan. He or she can spend money, or make investments only according to what the court authorizes. Another order from the judge is required before any changes can be made to the plan. Whether or not the committee also has authority over personal rights varies from province to province.

Committeeships are generally expensive. The committee has to be bonded by an insurance company and has the right to be compensated for administering the estate. Often, though, if the committee is the spouse or a relative, the right to compensation is waived. Sometimes the Public Trustee also waives compensation if it is evident that there are financial difficulties. Annual passing of accounts in court is usually required.

MAKING A WILL

If your family member with Alzheimer Disease has never made a will, you should encourage the making of a will while the person is still aware and can make reasonable and sound decisions. This is very important for two reasons. It will ensure that your family member's wishes will be carried out after death, and he or she will not die *intestate*, which means that all the assets of the person will be divided among the survivors according to the specific law of each province. Also, if the ill person waits too long, there is the possibility that the validity of the will could be contested, since it could be said that judgment was impaired as a result of Alzheimer Disease. The will should be drafted by and signed in the office of a lawyer.

Your own will should be reviewed carefully with your lawyer. There are several issues to consider. You may have left your entire estate or part of your estate to your family member with Alzheimer Disease. Or, you may have named the Alzheimer patient as executor of your estate. Since he or she will not be able to handle these responsibilities in the future, you should consult with your lawyer about what changes to consider and how to go about making them. You want to ensure that you have made provision for the care of your relative if you die and that other family members have access to your wishes and instructions.

The same points that applied to who should be granted power of attorney, apply to who should be the executor of your estate. You can have more than one executor at the same time, and should name an alternate if only one executor is named. As with an attorney, the executors should be geographically accessible, completely financially trustworthy and responsible, and if more than one, they should get along with each other.

An *Inter-vivos Trust* may be loosely described as a kind of will–a living will that takes effect while the person who makes it is still alive. This kind of trust document is sometimes drawn up when there is a particularly large estate. Ask your lawyer to advise you about the appropriateness of this trust document to your situation.

FINANCIAL MATTERS

If an Alzheimer patient owns or runs a business, you might find that the person is unable to keep up and you may need to think about some options.

Harry had owned a small hardware store for many years. His customers counted on receiving personal service. They often asked questions about the quality and reliability of certain products and depended on my husband's knowledge of his business. As the disease progressed, he started to have difficulty keeping up with customer inquiries. He became irritated easily, and then felt frustrated that he had lost his temper. Sometimes he forgot to place special orders and the other salesman had to step in to cover up for my husband's mistakes. It was the salesman who came to me and suggested that something would have to be done.

You may be able to find someone to help run the business for awhile, such as some of your children, other relatives, or a close family friend. You may be able to hire someone to help with the business. If none of these alternatives are viable, you may need to sell the business. Involve your ill family member in this decision, so that he or she will understand what is happening and why.

If you delay in selling the business too long, you will not get as much money if the operation starts to deteriorate. If you can sell it as a thriving concern, and the new owners can take over easily, you have a much better chance of getting the best price. Always seek experienced legal advice before signing any contract to sell a business.

Although you may be tempted to keep the business as long as possible so that your family member feels busy and useful, there may be negative financial repercussions as a result of waiting too long. Here are suggestions for alleviating this problem.

1. Make your family member feel useful by involving him or her in selling the business (this will also prevent undue suspicion and mistrust on the part of your family member).

2. Find some volunteer work or part-time work that your family member can pursue. This will not be easy, but might be worth the try.

3. Find some work at home that will give your spouse a sense of responsibility and usefulness as long as possible; for example helping with household chores. The person could fold laundry, stack mail, or help you dry dishes.

Since selling a business may be a very difficult step for an ill family member, do not give the option of *whether* the business should be sold. You may find yourself in an argument that is irrational and goes nowhere. Instead, be definite about the decision and involve the person. For example, you can say, "We are selling the business and we are going to the lawyer to sign papers." If you're going to sell the business, get power of attorney and use it if necessary.

A PARTNERSHIP

Your family member may be in partnership with one or more people. In that case, there will likely be a partnership agreement or a shareholders' agreement that will provide for the obligations of each partner in case someone wants to opt out of the business, or if a partner is mentally incapacitated. Consult your lawyer about this situation.

ROUTINE FINANCES

1. Money and Credit Cards. If your family member has credit cards, it is possible that irrational purchases will be made, since loss of ability to judge and reason accompany Alzheimer Disease. We recommend that you prevent this from happening by ensuring that these cards are destroyed.

    You may want to leave a small amount of money in the Alzheimer patient's wallet since spending this can't do any harm, and may help to give the person a feeling of reassurance and normalcy. It can be part of a person's identity to have some money in a wallet or purse.

    You may find that your relative seems overly concerned and preoccupied with money, and asks to go to the bank constantly, or wonders where the money is, or asks for money repeatedly. It might help if you reassure the person that there is enough money for the care she or he needs.

2. Bank Accounts. If you have a joint bank account that requires only one signature, only your signature will be required to transfer funds to an account in your own name so that you can administer your spouse's funds (some joint accounts–usually business accounts–require two signatures).

3. Old Age Pension and Canada Pension. You will be able to obtain an application to Health and Welfare Canada to have cheques paid to the caregiver in trust for the person with Alzheimer Disease.

4. Income Tax. We recommend that you consult with a chartered accountant to find out about deductions for which you may

qualify because of your relative's condition. It will be helpful if you record and keep careful track of expenses you incur such as medical bills, homemaking help, and other services you require as a caregiver.

Make sure that the accountant you choose is familiar with dementia and is someone with whom you feel comfortable discussing your financial situation. If you do not know a chartered accountant, use the same networking strategy to find one as you used to find a lawyer. Ask friends for a referral or check with your local Alzheimer society. Remember to check the fees.

Other issues you will want to discuss with the accountant include Registered Retirement Savings Plans, and any stocks and bonds that your family member may own.

5. Insurance Policies. You will need to review the terms and conditions of any kind of disability insurance your family member may have to see if he qualifies for benefits. See a lawyer with insurance experience if a claim for group disability insurance is denied under a disability policy.

6. Company Benefits. Check with your lawyer and the advisor of your family member's company about the status of any company benefits including profit-sharing, pension and retirement plans, and savings plans.

THE BENEFITS OF EARLY PLANNING

In this chapter, we have identified some of the legal and financial issues that may need your attention, and we have explained how to obtain the necessary resources. On legal matters, it is important to act early in the course of the illness for the following reasons.

1. You need the participation of the Alzheimer patient in the legal and financial planning process. In the early stages an Alzheimer patient can understand the meaning of your discussions and your financial and legal actions.

2. You may not know where the ill person has kept certain documents, receipts, and files that pertain to your financial and legal situation. Before your relative's memory is too impaired, you should check where items such as bank books, ledgers, insurance policies, savings bonds, and employment records are located. When you have located these, lock them in a special file drawer or container to which you have access. The Alzhei-

mer patient should not know where they are since he or she could throw them away, lose them, or damage them.

3. Acting early will give you peace of mind and allow you to direct your energies to the changes in your lifestyle. As the disease progresses you are bound to be under more stress, and it will be more difficult for you to think clearly about financial and legal matters.

To help you plan, you could make a list of things you need to do. Your legal list might look something like this.

1. Call Chairperson of Alzheimer Family Committee for referral to lawyer.

2. Call lawyer's office for appointment.

3. Check fees of lawyer.

4. Make list of issues and questions that need immediate attention, such as power of attorney, and making of a will.

5. Call a family meeting if possible and appropriate, to discuss the plans.

Beside each item, write down who will do the task. You could ask a friend or relative to make the appointment for you and help you with your list of questions so you are not overwhelmed with what has to be done. Use your personal support network to share the load and ease your caregiving responsibility.

FURTHER READING

Alzheimer Society of Metro Toronto. *Alzheimer's Disease: Legal and Financial Concerns–Revised Edition.* 1984.

Levin, Nora Jean, *How to Care for your Parents: A Handbook for Adult Children.* Washington: Storm King Press, 1987.

7

WHAT WILL HAPPEN
TO YOU?

❧

It is difficult to be a spouse, relative, friend, or lover of someone with Alzheimer Disease. It can be a long illness during which the person you once married, confided in, shared with, and loved, looks physically well and the same as before, but is different in mood, behaviour, and ability to think and remember. Coping and caring in the best way possible are accompanied by grieving for the loss of the person you knew.

A CHANGE IN YOUR EMOTIONS

Alzheimer Disease affects not only the person with the disease, but also all the members of the family. Throughout this book, we refer to you as a relative of someone with Alzheimer Disease, and as a caregiver. You are also still a separate person and you have feelings.

This chapter articulates the changes you can expect in your personal life–how you will feel, differences in your social relationships, and causes of stress. You will find out how to gain a degree of control of these changes; when you need help; and how to get that help.

ANGER: WHAT TO DO ABOUT IT

I resent not being able to share my days and my life with my husband.

I get frustrated and angry at having to repeat things over and over and then I feel guilty at showing my anger.

It makes me angry to have to depend on so many other people to help me with my wife.

I am angry that my wife is sick and I am helpless to make her better.

You may find it difficult to accept feelings of anger and frustration. After all, you have a husband or a wife who is sick; it is nobody's fault; and still you get angry with the person for forgetting things, or for embarrassing you. You resent not being able to carry out plans you made together for the future. You may be thinking, "What kind of person am I to react this way?"

The answer is that you are normal. It is usual and legitimate to feel angry. Accepting that you have a right to feel angry will help relieve the feeling of guilt, and will help you find ways to deal with your anger.

Dealing with this anger is difficult, because keeping it inside can be harmful to you, but expressing it openly can cause confusion, disorientation, and can hurt the person you love. Your relative will not understand the cause of the anger, but will sense your angry tone and look.

Some people who have been close to an Alzheimer patient suggest the following ways of dealing with anger.

1. Talk to friends about how you are feeling. Having an opportunity to express your anger to someone who understands can be an effective source of relief for you. You could talk over the telephone, or meet with a friend. Choose someone you are close to and who understands the situation.

2. Put your anger on paper. Some people find it helpful to let out their anger in the form of a letter to a friend or relative. Often, once the letter has been written, they feel better and don't actually need to send it. Other family caregivers find it extremely useful to keep a personal journal of their feelings and experiences. Recording your feelings in a journal will help to get them out of your system without upsetting the person who is ill.

3. Go for walks or engage in other physical exercise or physical work that you enjoy. The physical effort required will help to dissipate some of your feelings of anger. Often this kind of activity will give you a chance to get a different perspective on the situation and will allow you to return to your sick relative feeling better. If you are unable to go out, find a job around the

house that requires physical activity such as baking, or cleaning, or rearranging cupboards.

4. Attend an Alzheimer family support group on a regular basis. You will find support and practical suggestions from others who are and have been experiencing the same feelings. The mutual support group can be a safe place for you to discuss what is making you angry and why.

5. Try relaxation techniques. Some caregivers find that relaxation techniques such as stretching exercises, relaxation tapes, Tai Chi, or yoga can be effective. Yoga and other stretching classes are offered by many community centres and continuing education programs. You could ask your family doctor to recommend some relaxation techniques.

GUILT: IS IT MY FAULT?

You may find yourself wondering whether you are responsible in some way for your family member's illness. You may be asking yourself if Alzheimer Disease could have been prevented. Perhaps you worry that you pushed the person too much, or that you made too many demands. You may wonder about the diet of the Alzheimer patient and whether this had something to do with getting the disease. You may feel guilty about past events in your marriage and your life together that cannot be changed now.

You are not responsible in any way for the fact that a family member has Alzheimer Disease. However, we know that feelings of guilt can be overwhelming and are hard to deal with. Even when you are reassured that you did not do anything that caused your family member to have Alzheimer Disease, you may find yourself still feeling guilty. It may help to discuss these feelings with close friends or relatives who know you well.

You may also feel guilty because you are well, and the person you love is sick. You are not alone. Many caregivers feel this way for awhile. It may help to share your feelings about this in a support group with others who are caregivers of a family member with Alzheimer Disease.

SADNESS: EXPERIENCING THE LOSS

One woman who joined a family support group after her husband had been diagnosed with Alzheimer Disease for several years expressed her feelings this way:

I feel like I've been grieving for three years. I still love him, but he is not the same person I married and lived with for thirty-two years. I miss my husband. It's hard to remember him when he was vital.

You have reason to feel sad. You are experiencing the gradual loss of a loved one. You may also be feeling sad because of the loss of the dreams you shared for the future.

Some family members report that they feel like they are mourning even though the person with Alzheimer Disease is still alive. Grief is not something that is experienced only following a death, but is an emotional reaction to the experience of loss. Mourning is the process that allows a person to incorporate the loss into the present life. In general terms, the mourning process can include initial shock, intense emotional expression, experiencing loneliness, and finally, establishing new relationships.

The key word is process, something that takes time. You need to allow yourself time to absorb the changes that are happening to you and your family member, and to adjust.

Some signs to watch for that indicate that your feelings of sadness, depression, or grief are interfering with your daily functioning include the following.

1. Change in eating patterns. You may notice that you no longer have an appetite and have lost a lot of weight as a result; or you may notice that your weight has increased and you are eating more than you usually do.

2. Change in sleeping patterns. You might find that you are waking very early in the morning, not sleeping very well at night, or sleeping much more than usual.

3. Lack of energy. Are you feeling tired and listless most of the time? Is it difficult to maintain an interest in activities and people around you?

4. Inability to concentrate. It might be increasingly harder for you to focus on what you have to do each day, or on what you are reading. Your usual ability to pay attention to a speaker, watch a television show, or remember details may be reduced. You may no longer be able to find pleasure in activities that require concentration.

5. Mood changes. You may notice that you are crying a lot or more than usual, and that you are much more irritable with family members and friends.

6. Hopelessness. You may find that you are feeling hopeless about the future most of the time. You may also feel lonely and isolated, despite the presence of friends and relatives who could help. These feelings of despair may lead to anxiety and even to thoughts of suicide.

CONSULTING A PROFESSIONAL HELPER

If your usual ways of handling your anger are not working, or if your feelings of guilt, sadness, and depression are lasting a long time and you are experiencing the symptoms described in the above section of this chapter, you may want to arrange to see a professional therapist.

Use your network to help you. Start by discussing with your family physician how you have been feeling, or with your clergyman if you have a close relationship with him or her. These people may be able to provide the perspective you need, and help you feel better.

If they cannot help you, ask them for a referral. Examples of the kind of professional who could help include a social worker, psychologist, psychiatrist, or nurse. When you are asking for a referral, remember to find out what the fees are, and if your medical insurance covers the cost of this counselling.

Remember that you should be comfortable with the therapist you choose. If you feel that you are not being helped, it is all right to ask for another referral. You need to talk to someone who understands dementia and your role as caregiver.

Going to a professional counsellor or therapist is another part of building a network of services. You may need this kind of professional help for only a very short period of time, but you will know that it is available for you if you need it again in the future.

A CHANGE IN YOUR PARTNER
RELATIONSHIP

The relationship you had with your partner, the role you played as husband or wife, and your social relationships will change as you live with Alzheimer Disease. These changes will be a source of stress for you and your whole family. Knowing generally what to expect will help you to prepare. Remember, though, that each person's situation and relationships are unique. The suggestions in this chapter need to be applied in the context of your individual situation.

PRACTICAL MATTERS

As a partner in a marriage and in a family you have certain ways that you organized the work in your household. Living with Alzheimer Disease means that you may have to take on new jobs that are unfamiliar. For example, the bookkeeping and finances, the invest-ments and the banking may have been things your spouse who is now ill managed alone; or perhaps you both shared these tasks. Now these may become your sole responsibility. This may be overwhelm-ing and cause you to feel inadequate.

> My wife was the one who always looked after buying the grandchildrens' Christmas gifts and remembering family birthdays. The first time I had to think about making a gift list and shopping for presents was overwhelming for me. My daughter-in-law offered to take me shopping and gave me hints about what to buy. It felt lonely to be doing something that my wife had always managed so well.

Family social events and planning activities with the children may always have been the responsibility of your spouse. Perhaps your mate was the one who repaired a light switch or a leaking tap, or managed the daily running of the house, including shopping, laundry, and homemaking in general.

Taking on new roles, especially in time of stress, is difficult. It may make it easier to develop an action plan. For example, if you have never learned about banking and investment procedures, your action plan might look like this.

1. Speak to the bank manager and explain the situation to him. Ask for an explanation of what you must do and how to streamline banking procedures.

2. Speak to the accountant about what has to be done on a monthly and yearly basis, and how best to ensure that all bookkeeping matters are looked after.

3. Get help from a relative or friend who might be able to make bank deposits or pay bills. (Another alternative would be to obtain the services of a respite-worker to stay with the Alzhei-mer patient while you do the banking.)

4. Simplify current arrangements. (For example, you may need to centralize several bank accounts into one location so that you will have to make only one trip to the bank.)

You feel more positive and in control if you make a list of all of the tasks your ill relative can no longer assume and then formulate action plans for dealing with them. The action plan will identify who you can talk to, and how the task can be handled.

If you and your spouse shared most roles and responsibilities, you will feel the pain of carrying on by yourself. Finding ways of getting help will make these activities less lonely.

Remember that if your relative is still able to assume part of a task, it is important that she or he participate to the maximum degree possible. For example, if making a deposit is too difficult, perhaps the person can go to the bank with you and hand the completed slip to the teller. Try to find a balance between helping the person maintain self-esteem and having unrealistic expectations.

YOUR INTIMATE LIFE

You may find that the relationship you had as husband and wife, lover and friend, is now changing into one of caregiver and patient, giver and receiver of care. In the early stages of the disease this may not be as noticeable. As you become more and more responsible for decisions that have to be made and as your spouse becomes more dependent on you, you will feel the change more acutely. You will miss the equal sharing with your partner.

Although you may be able to continue to share thoughts, plans, and experiences in the early stages, this will become impossible as the disease progresses. If your marriage was a close one characterized by intimate sharing, you will feel this even more acutely.

Changes in the way you relate sexually to each other may be very stressful for you. Although your partner may still need and want to make love, you may find this difficult because of the other ways your relationship has changed. Not being able to exchange opinions, feelings, and ideas on an intellectual level may make sexual sharing awkward and uncomfortable for you.

This is a very personal subject and not all friends or relatives will be comfortable if you confide in them about it. In fact, not all counsellors are comfortable or effective dealing with this kind of personal issue. You should recognize that it is a very legitimate problem, not one that you need to hide or feel too embarrassed to discuss. Your family physician may be helpful, or may refer you to a therapist who specializes in marital therapy and who will understand the sexual problems accompanying dementia.

Use your network to find a professional helper you feel comfortable talking to. You can change therapists if you need to without feeling guilty or embarrassed.

NEW RELATIONSHIPS

Some family caregivers are able to form new relationships either while the Alzheimer patient is still at home, or after placement in an institution. The pleasure that this brings is often accompanied by guilt and uncertainty. Some caregivers are very comfortable with this concept; others wonder whether it is legitimate to enjoy a new friendship and perhaps a sexual relationship under these circumstances.

Every person's situation is different, but remember that a basic premise of this book is that you are a person as well as a caregiver. The key is to find ways of enjoying a new relationship that will work for you.

> My aunt met someone at a support group with whom she felt comfortable and at ease. They started to go out for coffee sometimes after the meeting. At first their friendship was based solely on their common experience as caregivers. Gradually, they started to go to a concert or movie together. It was only after my uncle was in a long-term-care facility that the family ever met her new friend. At first, only a few relatives knew about the relationship. Once my aunt felt that her new friend was accepted by them, she was able to bring him to more family social occasions.

CLAIMING YOUR HISTORY

You may be able to ease the stress of not being able to share by reaffirming the past and what you still mean to each other. It may help to keep in touch with close friends who knew you and shared experiences with both of you together. They will understand when you talk about what you are missing. Memories of shared past events, trips, and experiences with relatives and friends who knew you and your spouse may help you to claim your history.

You may want to make an appointment to talk to a professional who knows you both and who shares history with you. This could be your family physician or favourite clergyman. Try looking at family photographs together, and with other relatives and friends, or in a quiet time by yourself to reaffirm the history of your relationship. Some family caregivers find it extremely helpful to write a history of past events that have significance and that can be reclaimed through writing, reading, and sharing with others.

UNFINISHED BUSINESS

There are often thoughts in a marriage or a relationship that are important but are unspoken. You will not be able to speak to your family member about these things once the disease has progressed past the early stages. If you are able to find a way in the early stages of the disease to discuss personal issues, decisions, experiences, or feelings this will likely give you peace of mind later.

You might lead into your discussion of unfinished business by looking at old photos and reminiscing. This will make it easier to approach the issues and feelings that need to be talked about and shared. Once you have initiated the discussion, your partner may wish to bring up some things as well. Remember that concentration may already be a problem, so try to keep the discussion simple and focused.

SOCIAL ISOLATION

There are friendships you and your partner will have developed that include people who come to visit, people you go out with on a regular basis, and people with whom you attend a regular club, organization, or social or religious organization.

You may find that your social relationships are shrinking. Your partner will no longer be able to play cards or other social games that require concentration. This is difficult for other couples to tolerate. Unless they know you very well, they may hesitate to include you both when planning this kind of social time. It will also be difficult for your partner to engage in social conversation and small talk and this may make others feel uncomfortable and self-conscious. Your partner's behaviour, either at home or while visiting, may be unpredictable and this also can cause embarrassment to friends and acquaintances.

The number of activities you were able to do together will decrease as the illness progresses. It will be difficult for your partner to follow the plot of movies or plays as concentration and memory skills are lost, and music may only sound like loud noise.

My husband and I used to look forward to concerts—string quartets were his favourite. We were sitting in the front row at the last concert we attended when my husband suddenly yelled out "stop all that noise." We left quickly and I cancelled our subscription after that incident.

You owe it to yourself to pay attention to your own needs for friends and social and cultural activity. Try a combination of the following solutions to the problem of shrinking social relationships and activities.

1. Use respite services or informal helpers to give you time to maintain friendships and social activities outside of the home. Respite services are discussed more fully in Chapter 5.

2. Develop new contacts through the Alzheimer Society. You will meet people who understand what you are living, people who have been there themselves.

3. Seek out one or two friends or relatives with whom you have always felt the most relaxed and comfortable and invite them over on a regular basis. The consistency will help your partner adjust to the company, and your friends will become used to unusual behaviours.

4. Consider saying yes when you receive invitations to a friend's for dinner. Do not automatically refuse. If your spouse cannot manage the occasion, go yourself even though it may feel awkward at first and you will probably worry about your partner while you are out.

5. When you don't feel like talking or listening to people, you still may feel less isolated if you go out where there are people around. Going to the library, or a movie, or a shopping mall may make you feel more "normal"; activity surrounds you but these places make no demands on you.

6. Allow yourself to stay connected with people and activities. If you are used to going to an exercise class once a week, or used to like to see a play with friends, try to find ways to continue even if it is not as often as before.

7. If you have always wanted to learn macrame or try vegetarian cooking, it might be a good idea to find a course. Avoid trying to learn something that is taxing, however, because your purpose is to relax in this new activity, and not add to the stress you are already experiencing as a caregiver.

8. There is no reason to feel guilty for taking time for yourself. You deserve it and, besides, it will not help your spouse if you become too run down or depressed to give the best care you are capable of providing. You will return to your caregiving role healthier and more refreshed.

ADULT CHILDREN: ISSUES AND OPTIONS

My father has Alzheimer Disease but right now I feel like the biggest problem is my mother. She insists on playing the martyr and it is a real battle to get her to take a break and allow others to give her a hand. I am worried that soon there will be two patients. My brother and sister live out of town and are sympathetic, but removed, from the immediate situation. We have a small child. It is so hard having to take so much responsibility for what is happening.

One of the themes of this book has been that Alzheimer Disease affects the whole family. The role of the adult child or children needs special attention.

THE BALANCING ACT

Juggling your needs, the needs of your own family, and the needs of your parents at this time can seem like an impossible balancing act. You can put some perspective on your responsibility if you use some of the resources for community help identified in Chapter 5, and some of the skills in Chapter 8.

1. Become aware of available community resources and services in your neighbourhood and in the community so that you can be in a position to provide informed advice to your parents.

2. If it is possible, organize a family conference so that tasks and responsibilities can be shared with other siblings and close family members. This will also help to reduce stress by ensuring that there is consistent communication among family members concerning what is happening and why.

3. If a family conference is not possible, make a list of tasks that have to be done. Activities that seem overwhelming in time and effort can be broken down into smaller steps. One family that we know of needed a live-in caregiver for their parent with Alzheimer Disease. They made a list of everyone in their network and shared the task of calling. They also decided to try an ad in the newspaper. They passed this record of their experience to another family:

- Write the ad. Newspaper staff will help you to word ads if you are in doubt about phrasing; look for other ads in the paper for live-in help and see what the usual wording looks like.
- Stress important priorities such as nursing experience, dependability, references.
- If you cannot receive calls all day place a time frame on the phone calls, such as "Call after 6:00 p.m. or before noon."

- Call one or two newspapers and find out which days are best for domestic ads.
- Compare costs.
- Place the ad.
- Screen callers over the phone to avoid having to interview too many people who are clearly not qualified for the live-in position.
- Insist on references that can be reached by telephone, and get details of past experience.
- Some agencies will answer the ad. Check their prices and conditions. You may want to try interviewing some of their clients if you cannot find a suitable candidate through your ad. The finders' fee may be worth the time and trouble you save in not having to place ads in the future.

4. Try to establish some consistent guidelines for when you can be reached at home or at work (not referring to emergencies). If you always have a staff meeting Monday at 10:00 a.m. or if you always take the kids to art class on Wednesday afternoon, make sure that your parents know this. This will help to set up consistent expectations. Your parent will be able to know how to schedule the respite-worker once he or she knows when you are not available to help.

5. You may find it helpful to participate in a support group either with your parent if he or she is comfortable, or by yourself. You may learn how other busy family members in your position handle the situation, and you will have a chance to express your feelings and obtain support.

6. You may have to become the case manager or the co-ordinator of care for your parents. This can be time consuming and frustrating unless the key people such as homemakers, physicians, and social worker, are accessible to you. Be sure that you have their names and phone numbers, and let them know what you are doing and that you should be kept informed of changes or their concerns.

   If you are being asked to play the role of co-ordinator or case manager and cannot fulfill this responsibility, inform the key people so that expectations are clear and other ways of co-ordinating services can be found.

7. It will become increasingly difficult to include your parents in

events outside of the house. Some trade-offs may be necessary. You could try to take an event to your parents. Hold a birthday party at their place instead of at the usual restaurant. This may mean compromises in the number of people you invite and in the kind of party activities.

On the other hand, you may decide that it is very important to your family to have the event in the restaurant as planned. You could arrange for your parent who does not have the disease to come for part of the time while someone stays with your affected parent.

Trade-offs between the needs of your own family and life and those of your parents will have to be made on a case by case basis, taking into account the number of people involved, the uniqueness of the occasion, the type of event and the intensity of feelings.

CHANGES IN A PARENT'S MARRIAGE

Some adult children find it hard to accept the fact that the parent who is the caregiver has formed a new relationship. They often feel their parent is being disloyal. Others are relieved that their parent has found a new companion.

How you react and how much of your reaction you share and express to your parent is a very personal decision. You might find it helpful to share your concerns in a support group where other adult children have experienced similar feelings and reactions.

My father had Alzheimer Disease and lived with my mother in another province. I was dreading my visit because my mother had been depressed and I wasn't sure I was up to helping both her and my father. She met me at the airport and told me on the way home that she had met a new friend. She wondered if I wanted to meet him during my visit.

I should have been relieved that she seemed less depressed and much happier than on my last visit. It surprised me to find that I was upset that she was going out with this new person and that I was uncomfortable about meeting him. I decided that my reaction was my problem and not hers. Although I managed to find an excuse to not meet the new friend, I did not express any disapproval or concern during my visit.

FURTHER READING

Tanner, Frederika and Shaw, Sharon. *Caring: A Family Guide to Managing the Alzheimer's Patient at Home*. The New York City Alzheimer Resource Centre, 1985.
Zarit, Steven. *The Hidden Victims of Alzheimer's Disease: Families Under Stress*. New York: New York University, 1985.

8

COPING SKILLS: HOW TO STAY ON TOP

❧

Alzheimer Disease is a family problem. It affects not only the patient but all the other members of the family as well. This chapter suggests ways to deal with the changes in mood and behaviour common to Alzheimer patients–to make the problems less burdensome, less traumatic for you as the caregiver, for the patient, and for other members of your family. The purpose of these suggestions is to help you carry out two major goals: to provide good care; and to give the Alzheimer patient the opportunity to function to the fullest capacity.

Sometimes these two things will be complementary. For example, you will feel you are providing good care when the patient is able to eat without help. However, sometimes it will be easier for you to dress the patient in the morning when you are in a hurry than for you to take time to lead him or her through all the small tasks necessary in dressing.

The ingenuity typical of an Alzheimer patient makes it impossible for us to identify and comment on all the things that might go wrong. Who would have imagined that a once-responsible person would put the garbage in the trunk of the car and put the groceries in the garbage? that he would hide the mail? or be arrested for shoplifting because he forgot to pay for the toothpaste?

Given this enormous variety of behaviour, we cannot tell you how to deal with every eventuality. We can, however, describe a series of skills that you can apply to whatever problems arise, to enable you to get through crises. Once you have mastered this set of problem solving skills, crises will seem less like crises and more like another vexatious wrinkle in an otherwise difficult day. As well, once you have come to understand the nature of the problem, and have worked out how to deal with it, you may feel comfortable about trying to anticipate a problem, and take action to prevent its recurrence.

> When I realized my husband was throwing out all the mail if he got to it before I did, I arranged for our mail to be delivered to our neighbours. Now I go over there, sort through the mail, put the important stuff in my purse, and bring home the junk mail for him to sort through.

This will help you begin to feel in control of your life, and that you are acting on behalf of your family member, rather than reacting to his unusual behaviour.

USE YOUR SENSE OF HUMOUR

Some people feel that a good sense of humour is the single most important coping skill you can develop. Being able to laugh when something would otherwise seem embarrassing, tragic, or enraging can help you carry on. It may even help you feel better physically.

You know the old saying, "I didn't know whether to laugh or to cry." We think you should laugh when you can. It's more fun, at least as good for you, and probably makes things better and easier for the sick person and other members of the family. Sometimes your laughter will help the patient, who may not know what you are laughing about, but will respond to the positive emotional tone of laughter better than to your tears or your anger.

Don't feel guilty about finding something funny. Laughing about something is not the same as laughing *at* someone. It is all right to find the particular behaviour funny. That is not the same as making fun of the person whose behaviour you are laughing at. Laughing gives you a physical and emotional release and helps put the behaviour into perspective.

Be careful, however, about sharing these funny incidents with other people, unless you know them well and trust them. Remember that if you tell them something funny, they will laugh. You need to think about whether you will feel comfortable about other people laughing at funny things your family member has done.

THINK IN TERMS OF TRADE-OFFS

Nothing in life–or in caregiving–is perfect. When you need to make decisions, it is often useful to think in terms of trade-offs, that is, think about what are the advantages and disadvantages of your alternative solutions, and how they weigh up against each other. Some people do this by making up lists with columns for Pro and Con. This may work for big problems, or problems that don't require an immediate solution.

Too often, however, you must make a caregiving decision on the spot. You do not have time to make all the lists when the bus for the day program is waiting outside and the Alzheimer patient refuses to put on his shoes. You will need to think about how long the bus will wait; whether you can send the bus ahead and take the person to the day centre later; whether forcing him to put his shoes on will upset him so much that he might as well stay home; whether the struggle over the shoes will spoil your day to the point where he might as well stay home; what you had planned for the day, and how it will affect your plans if you have to stay home all day; how much he enjoys and benefits from the day program and how he will feel later for having missed it.

Your thinking might go something like this: "The struggle isn't worth it. It is going to spoil my day and his day. I have nothing special planned for today. He might as well stay home since he is going to the day program again in two days anyway."

On the other hand you might say: "If I can just get over this shoe business, it will really be important for him to go since it's his only day for day program this week, and I have several appointments planned for myself."

As you read through the remainder of this chapter on coping skills, you will find some advice that seems contradictory. You will need to use the concept of trade-offs to decide what to do in given situations.

BE CONSISTENT BUT FLEXIBLE

Variety, they say, is the spice of life. But for a person with Alzheimer Disease, and for a caregiver, variety is an invitation to confusion.

Consistency is a most important principle for an Alzheimer patient. You need to be consistent with the past; although the person's mood and behaviour will change, his or her basic personality will not change. There will still be the same likes and dislikes, the same interests, and the same preferences.

Provide a consistent routine. Be consistent in your attitudes and expectations about the patient's behaviour. You should also try to have the same person or people giving care for your family member.

Despite the importance of being consistent and establishing a daily routine, it is important to be flexible when necessary. If, no matter what you do, a patient refuses to take a bath first thing in the morning, which is the usual routine, think about whether it is important enough to make an issue of it. Can you give him a wash in the sink now, and maybe convince him to take a bath later in the day? Is it possible to forego a bath all together for the day?

Routine and consistency are meant to make life easier for you and the person you are caring for. If you become so caught up in your commitment to them that you create other problems in the process, take a second look at your guidelines. Be flexible when that will make your life easier, as long as you are not jeopardizing your family member's health or safety.

ESTABLISH PRIORITIES

Providing good care requires that you be consistent in your behaviour and expectations, and that you know what your values are. Then you can decide what is important to you, and what you want to make a fuss about. To do this, you must establish priorities. For example, if you place a high priority on having your family member dressed a certain way, you may wish to choose his clothes for him. On the other hand, if the person's ability to act independently is more important to you than anything else, allow him or her to choose clothing for as long as possible.

The specifics of these decisions are not so important. What is importaaally establish your position on these
matters early on. This will save you time and trouble when decisions need to be made, and will help you be consistent in your behaviour.

Sometimes the trade-offs required in setting priorities are not as clear-cut as the question of who will choose what your family member will wear. Sometimes priority setting requires you to trade off basic issues of health and safety against the person's independence.

My wife was a gourmet cook, and she still liked to help in the kitchen. One afternoon I walked into the kitchen and found all the burners on. It killed me to have to take the fuses out of the stove, but I was really afraid she'd burn herself.

Sometimes you will have to choose between getting a job done and allowing the Alzheimer patient to do things for herself. You will need to consider your own time constraints, and external constraints, such as a doctor's appointment, or the arrival of a bus to take your family member to a day centre. Rushing a person through an activity can result in agitation. When there are time constraints, plan ahead, and provide support and assistance along the way, rather than having to rush to meet a deadline at the end.

BREAK TASKS INTO MANAGEABLE PIECES

This problem solving skill applies to tasks that the caregiver must carry out, as well as to tasks you would like your family member to perform independently.

Many of the tasks you may now view as overwhelming are ones you once handled easily. It is the extra stress of caregiving, and not a change in your abilities, that makes tasks now seem more than you can handle. Break your work into smaller, more manageable parts.

For example, suppose you decide to put name tags in the Alzheimer patient's clothes, in case he or she wanders away or gets lost. Thinking about getting the name tags and sewing them into fifty or sixty items of clothing may seem so impossible that you may decide to abandon the idea. However, if you make a list of small tasks, each of which is discrete, easy to accomplish, and moves you towards the ultimate goal, the task becomes do-able.

1. Make a list of places to call to see if they have name tags.

2. Depending on the size of the list, and the amount of time and energy you have, call at least one place on the list. Continue until you have enough information to make a decision. Your decision might be based on cost, whether the company will mail or deliver, and how quickly you can have them.

3. Order the name tags.

4. While you are waiting for them to come, make a list of which clothes you will put name tags in.

5. Decide who will put the name tags in. Do you want to do it yourself, or in the company of a friend? Or do you want to pay

someone to do it for you? If you want to pay someone, go through the same process of breaking the task down to determine how you will find someone to do the sewing for you. If you want to do it yourself, decide what is a reasonable number of name tags to sew each day.

Use the same approach in helping the patient to carry out a task. For example, the person may not be able to respond when you ask her to brush her teeth. To sustain her independence, you might help her with this job by breaking it into its individual pieces. How specific and detailed your instructions need to be will depend on how far the disease has progressed. In the earlier stages, for example, you may need only say, "Put the toothpaste on the toothbrush. Now brush your teeth. Now rinse your mouth."

As the disease progresses, you may need to include additional steps: "Pick up the toothpaste. Pick up your toothbrush. Take the cap off the toothpaste. Squeeze the toothpaste onto the brush. . . ."

ASSUME ERRATIC BEHAVIOUR MAKES SENSE

After washing his hands, Mr. Green threw the hand towel in the toilet, instead of folding it and returning it to the towel rack.

When Mr. Jones arrives home from work, his wife tells him that the housekeeper has stolen her wedding ring.

Mr. Smith continually asks to go to the bank at the shopping centre, even though his wife has told him they do not have an account there any more.

Each of these stories illustrates a behaviour that may initially seem irrational and bizarre. However, if we analyze them carefully, with a view to understanding the behaviour, we will see that each of them can be explained within the context of the world of the confused individual.

Mr. Green thought he was helping his wife by disposing of a dirty towel down the toilet. That was the best way he knew to get rid of things. Mrs. Jones wanted to protect her valuable wedding ring by putting it in a special safe place and when she couldn't remember where she put it, she assumed the housekeeper had stolen it. Mr. Smith's desire to go to the bank really reflects his own concerns about whether there is enough money to take care of him and his wife, a concern he does not know how to express in words any more.

Simply understanding that the behaviour makes sense, even if you don't yet understand it, may help you feel more tolerant of the behaviour. Actually, understanding the behaviour allows you to go one step further, and respond to the intent of the behaviour. For example, the next time Mr. Smith asked to go to the bank, his wife told him not to worry, that there was plenty of money to take care of all of them for a very long time. While Mr. Smith continued to ask to go the bank, Mrs. Smith felt in control of the situation, and Mr. Smith seemed to feel satisfied with her response.

There may be other explanations for the behaviours we have illustrated. The important thing is for you, as the person who knows your family member best, to find an explanation that makes sense, and that allows you to respond in an effective way.

> I want to go home.

> You wish that you were young again, and things made more sense than they do now.

VIEW DIFFICULT BEHAVIOURS
AS SYMPTOMS

The Alzheimer patient is not being difficult on purpose. Although the behaviour may hurt or embarrass you, this does not mean that the person has intentionally set out to do this. He or she may be feeling angry, hurt, frustrated, frightened or anxious, and uses the only means available to express these feelings. The difficult behaviour is a product of the disease, just like memory loss or loss of judgment. Knowing this does not necessarily make it easy to deal with. However, an awareness of where the behaviour is coming from should make it easier for you to distance yourself from the behaviour. Do not take the comments personally, and do not feel that your family member is "out to get you." Listen to the feelings under the words, and don't bear grudges from one time to the next.

> My aunt was a nice Victorian lady all her life, whose main goal in life seemed to be to keep things calm and peaceful. One day when I was visiting her, she tried to climb on a chair to get a teapot off the top shelf. As I went to stop her, she lashed out at me and called me a sonuvabitch. I was so surprised, and then I saw the humour in

this sweet old lady referring to anyone that way. My mother and I had a real giggle about it when I went home that night.

KEEP THINGS SIMPLE

People with Alzheimer Disease find it difficult to process too much information. Structure and routine make things familiar, and provide a frame of reference. Knowing he will always help with the dishes after breakfast gives the patient a routine to count on, and the familiarity of it may help him experience a sense of mastery and control.

Structure and routine will also help you, as a caregiver, because there is a plan for the day. The simplicity that a routine provides serves as a useful balance to the other stresses of caregiving, and will help offset the unpredictability of your family member's behaviour.

Do not, however, become so addicted to the routine that you forget that its purpose is to give you a sense of control; it is not meant to control you. Develop the ability to recognize when flexibility is more important than sticking to the routine.

Open-ended questions allow for more options than a person with Alzheimer Disease can handle. As the disease progresses, the number of options your family member can handle will decrease. If you ask the person what she wants to drink, she may not be able to respond at all, because she doesn't understand the concept of "drink" or because she can't remember the word for what she wants. Instead, you might present two options: Do you want tea or coffee with dinner? If that doesn't work, you may need to present only one option at a time, so that the person can answer each question with a yes or no. (Do you want tea? No. Would you like coffee? Yes.)

Never offer the patient a choice when he doesn't really have one. If a respite-worker is already at your house, don't ask your family member if he minds you going out, unless you are prepared to stay home.

USE A PLANNING GUIDE

To help you cope, the planning guide on pp. 100-101 summarizes the planning steps that you will have to take during the course of the illness and shows when you need to do them. The chart indicates when various planning activities should take place. However, just as there are no clear boundaries that separate the stages, so there are no absolute times for when different things should occur. What we have shown is the *latest* time to begin a particular planning activity. Because the course of Alzheimer Disease varies from one individual to another, you may want to do some of these tasks earlier than we have shown, but we do recommend not doing them later.

The chart shows that much of the planning should take place in the first stage, when caregiving needs are lightest. Because you will be providing the least amount of direct care in the early stage, that is when you will have the most time to deal with the kinds of planning in the chart. You will also be under less stress in the early stages, and will therefore have more physical, mental, and emotional resources to carry out early planning activities.

CAREGIVING AND PLANNING GUIDE

	EARLY (STAGE 1)	MIDDLE (STAGE 2)	LATE (STAGE 3)
Doctors Ch. 4	Get a professional diagnosis Choose/confirm family physician Make a drug record	Be a partner-in-caring working with your physician	
Talking about AD Ch. 3	Tell your relative Tell others: friends, neighbours, relatives, employer, shops		
Community Resources Ch. 5	Build a network Identify key persons, e.g.: —public health nurse —information centres —Alzheimer Society Identify kinds of service you will need, e.g.: —meals, homemaking, day-care, respite	Use check-list to choose appropriate services: day-care, respite Use home services as needed	
Informal Helpers Ch. 5	Build a network Identify key persons who can help, e.g.: —relatives, neighbours, friends	Stay connected with friends & activities to prevent social isolation Plan for new roles you will take on	

CAREGIVING AND PLANNING GUIDE (continued)

	EARLY (STAGE 1)	MIDDLE (STAGE 2)	LATE (STAGE 3)
Legal Issues Ch. 6	Choose/confirm lawyer Obtain Power of Attorney Review will Collect and store valuable papers		
Financial Issues Ch. 6	List assets Remove credit cards Review insurance policies Simplify bank accounts Choose/confirm chartered accountant		
Home Environment Ch. 13	Identify changes needed immediately and long term changes Call workers Get estimates	Make changes needed in home	
Emergency Planning Ch. 11	Designate someone to call in an emergency Find out if a long-term care facility has respite beds on an emergency basis		
Long-Term Care Ch. 14	Identify options available	Visit available options—use checklist Place relative on waiting list	
Staying Healthy Ch. 7	Watch for stress and signs of depression Use your network to get professional help if you need it		Planning for your future as a single person

FURTHER READING

Lyons, Walter. *Coping and Helping with Alzheimer's Disease.* National Advisory Council on Aging, 1984.

Mace, Nancy and Rabins, Peter. *The 36 Hour Day.* New York: Warner Books, 1981.

Powell, Lenore & Courtice, Katie. *Alzheimer's Disease: A Guide for Families.* Reading, Massachusetts: Addison-Wesley Publishing Company, 1983.

Springer, Diane and Brubaker, Timothy. *Family Caregivers and Dependent Elderly: Minimizing Stress and Maximizing Independence.* Beverly Hills: Sage Publications, 1984.

9

DAILY CARE ROUTINES

❦

This chapter gives you some suggestions for going through an ordinary day with an Alzheimer patient. The purpose of the chapter is to help you understand the kind of approaches to use in helping your family member function as independently and safely as possible.

GETTING UP

The day starts with your family member (and you) awakening and getting out of bed. If you remember the last time you woke up in the middle of the night and didn't know where you were, you can understand how the patient may feel on first awakening. A gentle reassurance and subtle orientation to remind him where he is and what's going to happen next should ease the person's transition into the day.

To help the patient get started, try to maintain a morning routine that is similar to the one the person had before her or his illness. If you used to go for an early morning walk together, continue that routine. If the patient always shaved and dressed before coming down to the breakfast table, let him continue.

Since different people have different daily rhythms, try to be sensitive and observe whether the patient naturally maintains previous rhythms. If she was a "morning person" before, it is likely she will still feel that way. If he is up and wanting to go and you hold him back, he may become angry and frustrated, which could precipitate a bout of difficult behaviour. Conversely, if a person was slow to start in the morning, respect that pace as well; rushing someone could also result in a behaviour problem. If the person's rhythm has changed as a result of Alzheimer Disease, you will need to adjust your approach to fit the change.

USING THE BATHROOM

In the early stages, the Alzheimer patient may not experience any difficulties in using the bathroom. As the disease progresses, however, she or he will require more and more assistance, and more and more reminders, about when and how to go to the bathroom. Eventually, you may expect the person to be unable to manage this function independently.

When your family member is having trouble using the bathroom, your first approach should be to try and discover why. The answer will affect how you manage the problematic bathroom behaviour.

Even though the average person does not think it through, using the bathroom requires a complex set of skills. First there is the cognitive task of interpreting the body feelings into the need to use the toilet, and either expressing that need to someone who can help or acting on that need oneself. Then, there are the physical actions of adjusting clothing, sitting down, cleaning oneself afterwards, rising from the toilet, readjusting clothing, flushing the toilet, and washing one's hands. Consequently, when someone has an accident, you must first determine which of the many skills is lacking.

To help you identify which skills are lacking and what kind of assistance the person needs, you might want to refer to Reisberg's model of seven stages. Reisberg proposes that skills are lost in the reverse order to which they are learned, and this insight might help you determine where the patient's deficits are. Reisberg also indicates that sometimes the borderline between one stage and another overlaps. This is only one guide to help you handle bathroom behaviour.

Using the bathroom also involves getting there in time, and being able to find it in the first place. If your family member is likely to have difficulty getting to the bathroom on time, try renting or buying a commode to eliminate stairs, long distances, and other impediments. Check with your local public health department about the possibility of obtaining a commode at a reduced cost, and about the option of trying it out to see if it is effective before you purchase one.

If you find that the patient is urinating in a way that is inappropriate but, in fact, *approximates* appropriate behaviour, that indicates that the person is still able to make the connection between the internal bodily feelings and the need to urinate, and that he or she can manage the physical skills. What then is going on? It may be that he or she cannot find the bathroom, or cannot get to it in time, or lacks the verbal skills to ask you to help him find the bathroom. Leaving the door of the bathroom open might help.

It is very important to establish and follow a bathroom routine, a schedule that you implement on a consistent basis. If you know that the patient always uses the bathroom first thing in the morning, two hours after afternoon tea, or one hour after lunch, anticipate the need by setting up a bathroom routine for these times. Even though this will not be fail-safe and there will be times when you will miss, at least you will reduce the number of accidents. If the person does have accidents, keep a record of the circumstances–the time, where you were, and anything else that may seem relevant–to help you identify a pattern that will prevent accidents in the future.

GETTING DRESSED

Getting dressed is a complicated process that involves numerous tasks that we tend to take for granted. One caregiver reported that she had to break the task down into eighteen different steps to help her family member get dressed by himself.

1. *Choosing Clothes* Clothes need to be appropriate to the weather and the activity. The patient should look well groomed and presentable. If the patient is still able to choose his or her own clothes, allow it even if *your* standards of taste are compromised. However, when the person can't choose, or can only make limited choices, then present her or him with simple options. The person should be allowed to continue to dress in the style that is familiar. Don't expect a woman who has always worn dresses to be comfortable in slacks; and someone who is used to wearing subdued colours won't suddenly feel good wearing bright ones.

2. *Putting Clothes On* Attention has to be paid to both the physical act and the cognitive act of dressing. Clothes have to be put on in the right order and in the right way, that is, not inside out or upside down. Then the physical finishings–buttoning, zippering–have to be accomplished. Reisberg's theory suggests

that people will lose the ability to select appropriate clothing before they lose the ability to put them on. This theory is described more fully in Chapter 12.

Dressing has to be broken into discrete tasks. One task may be as large as putting on a shirt, or as small as buttoning a button. Here is a really important place to focus on the skill the person still has, and to ask him to do those bits you know he can do.

3. *Buying Clothing* Buy clothing that is easy to put on and fasten. Pants and skirts with elastic waists eliminate the need for buttons and zippers. Velcro fastenings and snaps are easy to use, and elasticized clothing is easily available. Specially designed clothing for the elderly and the disabled is available in special shops. Look in the Yellow Pages, call an occupational therapist, or check with your local Alzheimer chapter to find out where you can buy these clothes.

Shoes should be comfortable and safe, especially if the Alzheimer patient paces. Just as we would expect continuity in the type of clothing preference, so too with shoes. A woman who has always worn high heels may not be comfortable in flats, but very high heels may not be safe. While loafers and moccasins are desirable because they are easy to put on and off and don't require skill with laces and buckles, some people may prefer the feel of a tied shoe. Shoes that close with velcro snaps give the security of a tied shoe without the problems. Don't encourage the person to wear slippers during the day. They are often not safe, and convey a non-verbal message that says the person is sick or non-productive.

Buy clothes that are easy to wash in the washing machine and don't require ironing. Do not buy clothing that needs to be dry cleaned. If the daily routine has become a bit messy, you may want to think about this for yourself as well.

MEALS

Meals are a very important part of the daily routine. As with other things, don't expect changes from the past. If the person didn't eat breakfast before the illness, this preference probably won't change now. It is the same with specific food preferences.

As long as the patient is able, and if you take safety precautions, encourage him or her to participate in meal preparation. Depending on the stage of the disease and the level of functioning of the patient, he or she could help with a major task like setting the table, or a smaller one like putting parsley on the turkey. As we described earlier, you may need to break down a complicated task into its smaller parts. It may be especially important to involve women in the preparation of meals, since some women think of kitchen and food as their particular domain and this is often an important part of their self-image.

The kitchen is often thought of and felt to be a warm and nurturing place. Encouraging your family member to help with activity in the kitchen will further this association.

Some aspects of having the patient help with food preparation can be frustrating. For example, one Alzheimer patient insisted on putting all the dishes in the cupboard after having helped to prepare a meal.

Another frustrating situation may occur when your family member forgets that he or she has eaten, and demands a meal. Instead of arguing, try offering the person a piece of fruit or some vegetable sticks and move away from the kitchen to another activity.

If the patient forgets to eat when he or she is alone during the day, or throws food away that you have prepared and left for him or her to eat, take note. This may alert you that the person cannot manage alone at home, and needs more help.

Mealtimes will be more pleasant for both you and your family and less frustrating if you follow these guidelines.

1. Reduce the choices that you offer at mealtime. Instead of two kinds of juice being available, or several salad dressings, provide only one. This will prevent confusion, and the difficulty of making a decision.

2. Serve only one course at a time. Otherwise, the person will not know which to eat first and may overlook one of the courses altogether.

3. Use seasoning while preparing food instead of leaving condiments on the table. An Alzheimer patient may lack the appropriate judgment to know how much salt and pepper to use. You also may need to ensure that the patient follows a special diet, such as low salt or sugar, and this will be difficult if salt and sugar are left on the table.

It will increase the sense of satisfaction your family member derives from a meal if you serve foods that are easy to eat without assistance. Examples include finger foods, vegetable sticks instead of a salad, and an egg sandwich instead of an omelette. When the patient is no longer capable of cutting food, try changing from beef to softer food like fish so that the person can still eat as independently as possible.

It is important for the patient to get plenty of fluids. Remember to check that drinks are not too hot since the person's judgment will be impaired.

Similarly, using plastic dishes and glasses will allow the patient to help you in the kitchen without a constant worry about dishes getting broken or your family member being hurt. Some plastic dishes and glassware are quite attractive, and it is worth taking the time to find some that you like, so that you can retain a pleasant feeling at mealtime.

Try to find some way to retain the dignity of the patient and at the same time deal with spills. A chef's apron, cobbler apron, or barbecue apron will help prevent spills on clothes with more dignity than a bib. If the person spills food on the floor, you may want to pick up the rug, if it is an area rug that is easy to lift. If you have carpeting, consider placing a plastic mat on the floor under the table, but be sure it is taped or tacked down securely, so that there are no loose or lifting edges to trip over. At the table, you can use plastic or straw place mats, since they are easy to wipe down. You could also use a plastic tablecloth, or a sheet of clear plastic over a regular tablecloth.

You may sometimes prefer to have an occasional dinner or lunch alone with music or a book after the patient has eaten. Allow yourself this treat since you will need the break from stressful meals. Give yourself permission to order in food once in awhile. It is a long day and you deserve it. Meals are good occasions to plan as outings with friends. Use respite-care services so that you can take advantage of this kind of social break.

You may also find that using prepackaged meals occasionally helps you. All meals do not have to be cooked from scratch. Pay attention to nutrition, but allow yourself to cut corners in food preparation. You can do this without jeopardizing the good nutrition and necessary vitamins that play an important role in good health for both you and the Alzheimer patient.

GROOMING AND PERSONAL CARE

The goal in personal care for the Alzheimer patient should be to encourage him or her to be as independent as possible and still be safe.

1. *Shaving* Use an electric razor. Remember, as with other tastes, if your husband never liked having a beard before, he won't now either.

2. *Hair Care* A simple haircut may be easiest unless your relative is used to something else and objects. It will be difficult to use rollers and styling brushes. Try to find a compromise that will still be attractive. This means not necessarily cutting hair short and straight like a bowl; long and straight can be easy to look after as well.

   If washing hair becomes a difficult process that causes upset, alternate the process with dry shampoo. Baby shampoo will help if getting soap in the eyes is a problem.

3. *Bathing* An Alzheimer patient may become resistant to bathing because the task seems too complicated. You can help by making sure the person really understands what a bath is and what you are asking him or her to do. You can use lots of non-verbal symbols, such as soaps and a towel, or point to the tub, to make sure the person really understands.

   Bathing should be a regular routine, done in the same way and at the same time as before the illness. If the person used to take a bath in the evening, don't suddenly expect him to take a shower in the morning.

   Bathing can be a dangerous activity, and you should supervise the patient even if she or he has been able to do this independently in the past. Check the water temperature (better yet, adjust the thermostat on the hot water tank). Make sure there is a rubber mat or decals in the tub and a properly positioned grab bar in the tub or shower. Be sure that whatever your family member will need (soap, washcloth, shampoo) is near at hand, so he or she will not have to reach or get out of the tub. If you leave him or her alone for awhile in the tub or shower, check in periodically to be sure the person is all right and that he or she is really washing. You might want to leave the bathroom door open, and stay nearby so you can hear if there are any problems.

   When the bath is over, make sure the person is dried well. If his or her skin is dry, after a bath is a good time to apply a moisturizing lotion.

   While the person is undressed for a bath is a good time to check the skin for sores and rashes. People who sit or lie down a lot may develop pressure sores that can be very painful and difficult to treat if they are left too long. These sores first appear as bright red spots, and are likely to appear on bony areas such as shoulders, elbows, knees, ankles and buttocks. Call the doctor if you find any evidence of these. He will give you something to treat them with.

As the disease progresses, you will need to provide more and more supervision, including making sure that your family member is washing properly. You may find that you would like a home care worker to assist the person with bathing; your family member may even find this less embarrassing than having someone in the family do it.

4. *Brushing Teeth* This may be a difficult task and you may have to break the task into smaller parts to help the person do it on his own.

Try to maintain a regular routine of brushing every day and alert the dentist if you find mouth sores. It is important that dentures fit properly since eating and nutrition may be affected, and your relative may not be able to tell you what is wrong.

Check whether teeth are really brushed, since sometimes the person with Alzheimer Disease forgets what brushing means and will say that it's done just to please you.

LEISURE TIME

Even with a structured day that has regular routines, there will be unscheduled periods. Leisure time is just as important to plan as structured time. Try to plan activities that the person enjoys. Include activities that you will also enjoy.

Exercise is very good, especially walking when the weather is appropriate. A certain amount of time spent watching television is all right, but there will come a time in the course of the disease when the person will no longer understand what appears on the screen. This will be frustrating and eventually television watching should be kept to short periods or curtailed all together.

You and your family member may also enjoy listening to music or just sitting. However, there may come a time when even music is difficult for the patient to understand and listen to, and it may be necessary to limit it to prevent frustration.

If the person always read a lot and enjoyed the paper and novels, he or she may still enjoy holding the book and turning pages. This can be a calming activity that is familiar and reassuring.

Try to relate leisure activity to hobbies that were important and enjoyable for the patient. Simple repetitive tasks will be easiest to handle. Examples include playing with a deck of cards, knitting (if the person remembers how to do it), sanding, if woodworking was a hobby. This is not the time to teach a new task or hobby.

> Mrs. Smith would only sit, rocking and moaning at home with almost no communication with others. One day she spotted knitting needles that someone had left and picked them up. As she remembered this former lifelong hobby, her rocking and moaning ceased and she was able to make increased contact with others.

People with Alzheimer Disease often have good long-term memory and enjoy reminiscing about the past. This may be a satisfying way for you and the patient to spend time together. Reminiscing gives the person a sense of continuity with the past, and will also give a sense of accomplishment.

Helping with household tasks can be a satisfying accomplishment and can help to maintain a person's self-esteem. It is also practical since it allows you to do your housework while you watch the patient. Although it would be faster in certain cases to do the work yourself, giving the patient something to do that makes her or him feel useful merits the extra time.

Try to select household tasks that are familiar. Men can adjust to helping around the house, and can help with activities such as collecting the laundry, emptying wastebaskets, and dusting. Folding laundry is a good activity to try since it is a simple repetitive task that has a satisfying textural aspect to it.

Sometimes you may be able to leave the patient alone with an activity, such as cards, and you may welcome the opportunity to finish another task on your own, or to take a break.

NIGHT-TIME

Sleep disturbances are common among people with Alzheimer Disease. Alzheimer Disease can make a patient restless and disoriented in the middle of the night, and unaware of the difference between day and night. Night wandering is one of the best known examples of sleep disorders. Sleep disturbances are among the most serious problems faced by family caregivers. Many family caregivers report that sleep disturbances are major factors that led them to move a patient to a long-term care setting. The loss of sleep robbed them of the energy needed to give care to the patient during the day.

Unfortunately, not enough is understood about sleep disturbance. However, just like other behaviour of people with Alzheimer Disease, some of these sleep disturbances do make sense. For example, often a person with Alzheimer Disease gets out of bed in the middle of the night to go to the bathroom but then does not remember where to go. You may have experienced this same kind of disorientation when you fall asleep on the living room sofa and then wake up and cannot remember where you are, or what time of day it is. Avoiding night-time fluids and diuretics will decrease the probability that a patient will get up in the middle of the night to use the bathroom.

If the Alzheimer patient does get up during the night and forgets he or she was asleep, you may find the person trying to get dressed, or in the kitchen getting something to eat. Gently remind the patient that it is still night-time, and that he or she can sleep a little longer before it is time to get dressed and eat something. You may have to compromise by giving the patient something to drink, and then lead him or her back to bed. Convey a sense of warmth and reassurance with a hug, a backrub, handholding, or even a drink of warm milk.

Try to discourage the patient from sleeping during the day, since this may reduce the need for sleep at night. Keep your family member dressed during waking hours. Providing activity and stimulation at a manageable level will keep the patient from sleeping because there is nothing else to do. Although you may be tempted to let him or her sleep while you do your chores or take a break, try to find another way of keeping the person occupied.

Some people have found that ensuring that a patient gets enough exercise during the day can be helpful in reducing sleep disturbances. The most common example is walking; dancing may also help. Going out in the car with you to the local shopping centre; carrying laundry up and down the stairs; vacuuming, or similar active tasks may also help. Remember, anyone who has spent the entire day sitting is unlikely to need a full night's sleep.

If none of these approaches work, you may wish to discuss the possibility of medication with your family physician or with a doctor who specializes in Alzheimer Disease. The use of sedatives may help a patient sleep, or they may cause hallucinations, nightmares, or otherwise increase disorientation. If you and your doctor decide medication is appropriate, you will need to monitor its effects carefully and keep your doctor informed of any problems that may arise, so the dosage can be adjusted.

If the sleeping problems are not otherwise controllable and you feel the loss of sleep yourself, you could investigate the possibility of paying someone to come and stay with the patient at night. (The need for care at night has been recognized by some groups that have considered providing "night-care" in a communal setting, as opposed to day-care. As of this writing, we are not aware of any community agency providing this service.) If the cost for night-care seems too high for you on a regular basis, consider arranging it intermittently.

If you have respite-care coming into your home, or if there is someone at your house during the day to assist you in caring for your family member, think about planning afternoon nap-time for yourself. This will help you conserve energy, and will prepare you for having to get up during the night with your family member.

Try changing your sleeping arrangements so that you are in a separate bedroom if possible, or in separate single beds. You may worry about not hearing the patient get up in the middle of the night. If you close the patient's bedroom door and put a bell on it, you will hear the bell when the door is opened. Make sure the bell you use is loud enough. One woman installed an electric eye beam across her husband's door; when he broke the beam by getting up during the night, a buzzer awakened her, and she went to his room to put him back to bed. Over time, the sounding of the buzzer came to be associated in her husband's mind with returning to bed, so that eventually when the buzzer went off he turned himself around and went back to bed.

Use night-lights in the bathroom and the bedroom to help prevent accidents at night. Some families have used reflector tape around the bathroom door to help a person find it.

FURTHER READING

Golden, Susan. *Nursing A Loved One at Home: A Caregivers Guide.* Philadelphia: Running Press, 1988.
Ontario Association of Homes for the Aged. *Guide to Caring for the Mentally Impaired Elderly.* Toronto: Methuen, 1985.

10
DIFFICULT BEHAVIOURS

❦

The changes in the brain that affect memory and judgment also affect the Alzheimer patient's behaviour. Some behaviour changes always accompany the disease to some degree. However, not all people with Alzheimer Disease will show all these problems, nor will they all occur to the same extent in everyone.

In this chapter you will find descriptions and reasons for some of the behavioural changes you can expect in a patient, and how to respond.

SUSPICION

You may find the Alzheimer patient accusing people of things that are totally unjustified. These suspicions may reflect the patient's inability to understand the world around him or her. Loss of memory and judgment prevent the person from developing appropriate explanations for things that are happening.

Often the accusations focus on things that your family member thinks have been stolen: a watch, keys, money, or a purse. When a person cannot find something, because memory is failing and they have forgotten where they put it, they think someone has taken it.

It's bad enough when you are the person being accused, but when the accusation is levelled at someone else, you may have to cope with resentments, anger, and hurt feelings. Simply assure the accused that you do not believe he or she is guilty of the "crime," and explain the reason for your family member's behaviour. This is all you can do.

SHADOWING

My husband follows me around wherever I go. He waits outside the bathroom door for me, and he drives me crazy.

It can be very distressing to be followed around all the time, especially since it is a constant reminder of how much the Alzheimer patient depends on you. Not only is your freedom to leave the house limited, but so is your freedom while you are in the house. Try to distract the patient by giving him or her something simple to do while you do your household chores.

ARGUING

Mrs. Jones asks her husband when they are going to have dinner. He tells her they have already eaten. She says she hasn't, she's hungry, and she wants dinner. He again tells her she has eaten, and he doesn't want to hear any more about it. She says she's hungry, and goes to the fridge to take out some food. He says she can't be hungry because she just ate, but she repeats that she is. Voices get louder, and both Mr. and Mrs. Jones simply become more frustrated and angry with each other.

This kind of situation can occur often in relating to any Alzheimer patient unless you have the skills to handle it. It's an easy trap to fall into, since the person still looks normal and healthy and often speaks with great conviction.

Pointless arguments contribute to a stressful daily living situation. It is difficult enough when people argue over things about which they truly disagree, but when a person argues with you about things that are as factual as whether or not you have had dinner, it can be extremely frustrating and draining.

Mr. Jones did not realize that although his wife had helped him prepare the meal, had enjoyed it enough to have seconds, and had helped him clear the table and dry the dishes, she did not remember any of this. In the absence of this memory, it makes no sense to continue an argument about past events. Knowing the cause doesn't prepare you for how to handle the situation, and pursuing the issue increases the frustration of both parties.

Even logic cannot be brought to bear on these situations, as the following incident shows.

At the end of the meal, Charlie asked where his tea was. Since he had just finished a cup of tea, his mug still felt warm and there was a slice of lemon in the bottom. When he denied having had the tea, his son pointed out the lemon in the cup. He agreed that he must have had some tea, but a minute later he again asked where his tea was.

Continuing with the argument leads nowhere. Instead, try to find a way to deal with the specific request that is being expressed. For example, in the case of the woman who forgot that she had eaten dinner, offer her some vegetable sticks and try to change the topic so that the argument is waylaid.

Another technique is to respond to the concern behind the words. For example, instead of arguing about whether or not your daughter visited yesterday, address the feeling that the patient would like to see her family more often. ("You miss Betty and wish she would come to visit. We'll phone her after dinner tonight.")

INAPPROPRIATE BEHAVIOURS

Inappropriate behaviours are those that cause you problems, that may appear irrational and bizarre, and can be embarrassing in the presence of other people.

I was so pleased when our neighbours dropped in; I really welcomed the relief. Suddenly my wife said "When are they going home?"

Our best friends had arrived for dinner, and we were waiting for my husband to join us. Suddenly he appeared at the top of the stairs without his trousers.

One of the best ways to deal with this kind of behaviour is to keep your sense of humour. It's not always easy to laugh, but do try to see the funny—even absurd—side of an Alzheimer patient's behaviour. If you are with people you trust and with whom you are comfortable, you might have a good laugh together. For your own sake, try to accept the reality that the Alzheimer patient cannot help his or her behaviour. There is no need to feel embarrassed by these unusual behaviours if everyone understands the nature of your family member's problem. It is important to explain the illness to everyone who spends time at your house visiting.

Try to be very straightforward and matter of fact in dealing with a given situation. Focus on the problem behaviour, and what needs to be done to fix it. If your husband doesn't have his trousers on, say "Excuse me, we have to go upstairs." The less embarrassed you are, the less uncomfortable and embarrassed other people will be.

Do not berate an Alzheimer patient for the strange behaviour. Remember that this behaviour is part of the disease, and is beyond the person's control.

Your relative's seemingly bizarre behaviour makes sense if you understand the context within which it occurs. If your husband formally introduces himself to someone he has known for many years, it may seem strange unless you realize that he does not remember seeing this person before. You can be better prepared to deal with the introduction if you consider the memory loss, and also if you have explained the illness to the family friend ahead of time.

You will not be able to anticipate every form of bizarre or unusual behaviour, so don't feel guilty about not having thought of something before it happens. On the other hand, notice the areas in which there are difficulties so that you will be better prepared for future occurrences. The next time an old friend comes to visit, you can say to your family member, "Isn't it nice that Fred has come to visit?" This subtle prompt will remind the patient of the friend's name without being obvious about the memory loss.

The kinds of unusual behaviours will change as the disease progresses, but the general approach to dealing with them will be the same. Later on, your husband may still have the ability to dress before coming to dinner, but table manners may have deteriorated instead.

AGITATION AND AGGRESSION

Sudden episodes of aggression can be one of the most disturbing behaviours for family caregivers. They are frightening for everyone, including the person with Alzheimer Disease. What is disturbing is not only the act of violence itself, but the feeling that the patient has lost control and is capable of punching, hitting, or pushing. Temper outbursts and loud screaming may also occur. This can be emotionally difficult to deal with, and can be especially hurtful when it is directed at you. Both these behaviours may seem to come quite suddenly and without warning, but they are not random, but rather the expression of anger, fear and frustration by an individual who has lost the ability to express feelings in more acceptable ways. These behaviours are usually set off in response to a specific incident or stimulus. Sometimes what sets off your family member may seem very trivial to you, but remember that if you lose ability even a small problem feels overwhelming.

You can help prevent these types of behaviour by being alert to factors that will lead to frustration and anger or cause fear. Don't push a patient to do things that are beyond his or her ability, and try to identify factors in the environment that may cause problems, even unintentionally. This will not always be easy, since what a person can do one day may be a source of frustration the next.

> My husband almost had a temper tantrum while he was trying to put on his shoes. He threw them across the room, and when I brought them back he hit me. Then I realized he was frustrated by the laces, and that afternoon we went out together and bought a pair of moccasins.

If an Alzheimer patient does become aggressive, try to remain calm. Your first response should be to protect your safety and the patient's, who may still be strong and able to cause harm. Your second step should be to calm the person and to reassure him or her. Remember that the Alzheimer patient is probably as frightened by his or her lack of control as you are by the aggression.

In dealing with agitation, the following steps should be helpful.

1. Try to remain calm, so that you do not add to the patient's distress. If you start yelling back, and the person senses your own anger, or fear, or frustration, he or she is likely to respond to it with increasing agitation. Ultimately, you increase the potential for a widening circle of upset.

2. If the agitation is directed at you, try to distance yourself and be objective about what is occurring. If your family member is angry or frustrated, remember that you are the only person to whom he can vent his feelings.

3. Focus first on calming the person. Use whatever techniques experience has taught you will reassure your family member that you are there to help, and that things will be okay. Some people will respond best to a reassuring touch or a hug. Make sure the person doesn't interpret this as an attempt to hold him or her down. Other people will respond best to a verbal reassurance. Often, the actual words you use matter less than the tone of your voice.

While a person is still agitated is not the time to try to address the cause of the agitation or the feelings behind it. In the midst of the upset, the person is unlikely to hear what you are saying anyway. Deal with the underlying causes of the behaviour after the patient has calmed down. If you can determine the cause later, you may be able to learn something that will help you in the future.

RESTLESSNESS

An Alzheimer patient may appear excessively anxious and show signs of restlessness. This may manifest itself in repeated pacing, rocking, and muttering. These can be extremely irritating, and will try your patience, especially when you may not be able to discover the cause.

Your first reaction, when this behaviour begins to bother you, may be to call the doctor to ask for a tranquilizer. In some cases, this may be appropriate, since the tranquilizer will alleviate not only the symptoms that you are having difficulty with, but also the underlying anxiety that is causing it. However, tranquilizers may impede the patient's ability to function, and you need to strike a balance between management and restraint.

You will need to be a partner with your doctor, and work closely with him or her to determine the appropriate dosage, and to monitor the changes in your relative's behaviour.

Before you call the doctor for medication, try these methods to alleviate the Alzheimer patient's behaviour.

1. Look for a pattern in these periods of restlessness. Do they happen at a particular time of day or in response to a consistent stimulus such as going to the bathroom?

   For example, if you notice that your relative has a bladder accident following a period of agitation, consider the possibility that this accounts for the restless behaviour. You can then structure a bathroom routine. Anticipating the cause of the restlessness will help relieve it, and give structure to the daily routine.

   Some staff in long-term care settings have identified a phenomenon they call sundowning, in which residents become particularly restless in the late afternoon. If you notice that this is also a time of restlessness for your relative, you may want to adjust the daily routine so you can plan an activity or pay extra attention to the person at that time of day. It may be an especially good time to go for a walk.

2. Try to redirect your family member into an activity that will channel the restlessness and energy in a constructive way. If he paces, think about taking him for a walk. If the person persists in repetitive behaviour with his hands, try an activity like folding towels, even if it means taking clean towels from the cupboard.

3. If you are anticipating a situation that may make the patient restless, such as a doctor's appointment where you may have to wait, plan ahead by bringing something with you that will occupy the person's time. For example, bring along a newspaper, even though the person may only hold it and not really read it.

WANDERING

When my wife wandered away she was missing for several hours. We finally found her on the other side of town. I can't imagine how she ever got that far, since her arthritis was so bad that some days she could barely walk from the bedroom to the living room.

One of the greatest worries of family caregivers is that the Alzheimer patient may wander away and get lost. This is a legitimate concern, and you must be prepared to deal with it even if you think it unlikely that your family member will wander.

Unfortunately, there is a great deal about wandering that is not understood. Even the reasons for it are not clear. In most cases, we believe, it begins as purposive behaviour, in that the person is looking for a particular place. Often the place being looked for is that symbolic "home" that people with Alzheimer Disease often refer to. In other instances, people may set off on what is to them a real errand–to the bank, the store, or to visit a friend–and forget where they are going and how to get there. Whatever the cause, the consequences can be serious.

There are two aspects of the wandering problem you need to deal with. One has to do with preventing the patient from wandering away; the other is how to increase the likelihood that he or she will be found quickly and returned to you if the person does wander away despite your best efforts to prevent it.

PREVENTING WANDERING

No matter how much you try, you cannot watch a person all the time. Therefore, you will need to modify the environment so that an Alzheimer patient cannot leave the house or grounds alone. This can be done by securing the door so that what the person must do to open it is beyond her or his physical or intellectual capabilities.

As there are several different types of locks that meet this requirement, you should probably consult a locksmith to determine which type will work best for your situation. If you contact the locksmith over the phone and explain the nature of the problem, he may be willing to come to your house and discuss the options with you.

There are several factors to consider in choosing a lock. First, what would happen if you had to get out of the house in an emergency such as a fire or explosion? In some jurisdictions the fire department may prohibit locks that make it difficult for you to exit the house in an emergency. Unless the rules clearly prevent it, however, you will have to decide which is the lesser problem: your family member wandering off or the difficulty of making a rapid emergency exit. Remember that it is unlikely that the patient would know what to do in an emergency even if there were no special lock on the door.

Some locks need a key to be opened from the inside as well as from the outside. This kind of lock may be an appropriate solution if you feel the patient would not be able to use a key. You can even hang a key near the lock for your convenience and for use in the event of an emergency, if you are confident that your family member will be unable to use it.

The simplest and least expensive solution is to put an additional lock or a sliding bolt at the top or bottom of the door. It is unlikely that the patient will think to look for a lock in these places.

Another factor to consider is the number of doors in your house, and where each leads to. If you are fortunate enough to have a door leading directly into a back yard, you may wish to secure it and make it easy for your family member to use this door for free access to the back yard in nice weather. When it is rainy or cold, you will want to limit the use of this door. The back door should have a lock that can be made inactive when you want so the patient can go between the house and the garden at will. A lock that needs a key to open it from the inside would be inappropriate in this instance.

To make the back yard secure, you must make sure that your family member cannot go out the gate or get out over the fence.

Because people with Alzheimer Disease have been known to show remarkable ingenuity and agility in climbing fences, the key to ensuring they cannot get over the fence is not to raise the height of the fence, but rather to make it more difficult to get to the fence by planting dense shrubs or bushes in front of it.

If you want to put a gate in the fence, you will need to use a mechanism that the patient cannot open from the inside. Something as simple as putting the latch on the outside, so that one must reach over the fence to open the latch, should be an effective solution to this problem.

WHAT IF AN ALZHEIMER PATIENT GETS LOST?

No matter how careful you are, it is possible that your relative may wander away from home, or may wander away from you in a public place. Even in the early stages of Alzheimer Disease, a person may become lost, confused or disoriented in a familiar place.

The following steps can increase the probability that your family member will be found quickly and returned safely to you.

1. Sew tapes with the person's name and address or phone number into his or her clothes. Remember that you don't have to sew them into all the clothes, because if the person is wearing pants she or he will likely also be wearing a shirt.

2. Have the patient wear an identification bracelet or necklace. Bracelets are preferable, since they are more difficult for a patient to take off. You can use a standard identification bracelet that you can purchase from a jeweller, or you can purchase a bracelet or necklace from the Canadian Medic-Alert Foundation. However, many people report that Alzheimer patients do not like wearing these bracelets and try to take them off. If you think your family member will take the bracelet or necklace off, or will hurt herself trying to get it off, you will need to look for another way.

3. In some communities, the police department has a program to register people with Alzheimer Disease. Check to see whether there is such a program in your community. If there isn't, and you have the time and energy, see if you can work with the police and the local chapter of the Alzheimer Society to set up such a program in your community.

4. Make sure you have a good, recent picture of your family member that you can give to police if you need their assistance

in finding him or her. Mark your family member's height and weight on the back of the picture.

5. Inform your neighbours and neighbourhood shopkeepers about the possibility that your family member may get lost. Give them your name and phone number, and ask them to call you if they see your relative out alone. If you live in an apartment building with a doorman, be sure to alert him to the problem.

6. If your family member goes out with another person, be sure that person understands that the patient must be brought home and inside the house.

You always hope your family member will not get lost. However, if he or she does, don't panic. The person may surprise you and get back home alone. It is best if you are there to calmly welcome him, so try to get other people out looking for him, while you await his return home.

FURTHER READING

Memory, Attention, and Functional Status in Community-residing Alzheimer Type Dementia Patients and Optimally Healthy Aged Individuals. *Journal of Gerontology* 39, no. 1 (1984): 58-64.

11
SPECIAL PROBLEMS

❦

Caregivers for Alzheimer patients encounter problems that often seem insurmountable: unpleasant social situations, travel predicaments, and dangerous driving when a person refuses to give up a licence. In this chapter you will find suggestions for solving these special problems and others unique to Alzheimer patients. Ideas on decision-making are included, along with some examples of other people's experiences.

If you have access to a family support group, you will find group members sharing their experiences of many of these problems.

DRIVING

The first big problem I had to deal with after my husband was diagnosed as having Alzheimer Disease was how to get him to stop driving. Even before the diagnosis, I had noticed he wasn't very safe on the road—he kept hitting the curb when he made right-hand turns—and I was getting nervous about driving with him. But he'd been driving for so long that it was like taking away a part of his identity when the doctor finally told him he couldn't drive anymore.

Convincing an Alzheimer patient that it is no longer safe for her or him to drive is a difficult task that many families must face. It's not always clear when an Alzheimer patient should stop driving. The diagnosis of Alzheimer Disease does not necessarily mean that the person should stop immediately. It depends on how advanced the disease is, and what faculties are still intact.

One way to decide is to *honestly* examine how you feel when you are riding with the person. Remember, your safety, the safety of your family member, and others on the road is at stake. Some people report that they do not like making the decision—they don't want to be the one to tell the Alzheimer patient to stop driving. Don't confuse making the decision with being the bearer of bad news.

Other families have said that even though they are worried about driving and their own safety, they do not want to take away what could be the person's last form of independence. Driving represents freedom, control, and a sense of mastery over the environment for many people. This is especially true for people who have been driving for almost all of their life.

There are also implications for you as a caregiver, especially if you have relied on the patient to be the driver. You may feel more isolated and alone if you are now the only driver.

Once you have decided that an Alzheimer patient should no longer be driving, you should discuss it with her or him. Tell the person firmly that you think he or she should not be driving any more. Explain why, and talk about what specific arrangements you will make. Here are some suggestions.

1. Establish a credit account with a local cab company. Keep credit chits available with the phone number for your family member to use.

2. If the person attends regular events such as a club meeting, arrange for another member of the club to pick up and bring her or him home. This arrangement is preferable to you driving the person since it is more "normal" to go with someone else than to be chauffeured by a family member. Just be sure the person who is driving understands the situation and knows the patient must be returned to the door of the house.

If you cannot convince the Alzheimer patient not to drive, ask your family physician to assume responsibility for telling the person.

This decision should be firm, and not negotiable. Families have found innovative ways to deal with the problem of preventing an Alzheimer patient from driving.

1. If you yourself do not drive, sell the car. However, if you would use the car to make life easier for yourself, we do not recommend this solution.

2. If you are keeping the car, the preferred solution is to park the car out of sight. Perhaps you can arrange with neighbours to use their garage or driveway. If necessary, you may have to rent space in another garage, or park on the street out of sight. This will prevent the frustration of the person seeing the car and not being able to drive it.

3. Some people have used other methods. These include hiding the car keys and locking the steering wheel. Some people have even resorted to removing the distributor cap. You could check with your mechanic about other ways of preventing the person from being able to start the car.

Having done all of this, you may still feel badly. This is natural, but it is far better than feeling responsible if your family member has an accident.

TRAVELLING

There are many different reasons why you might decide to travel even after your family member has been diagnosed as having Alzheimer Disease–to attend a social event out of town, to visit family members, or to take a vacation.

Whatever your reasons, careful planning will be necessary to be sure the trip goes as smoothly as possible. If you are flying, try to arrange your trip during an off-time when there will not be a rush of people so that processing tickets and baggage will be faster.

If you are going to an out-of-town social event, find out whether other people from your community or family will be attending, and if possible, arrange to travel with them. This will make the trip easier and more enjoyable for you, and there will be less need for leaving the Alzheimer patient alone.

To ensure the safety of your family member, be certain he or she is wearing detailed identification. In addition to the normal identifying information, be sure to include an itinerary, and a contact name and phone number.

If you travel by plane, take advantage of the early call to board. You may want to alert the airline to your problem when you make the reservation, and remind the flight attendant in charge of the flight.

Choose an aisle seat for easy movement, and a seat in the front section to prevent disorientation and distraction by the many other people. If the patient still reads, bring a book and also bring a deck of cards.

If you are staying in a hotel, we suggest a smaller hotel where you will have more quiet, and staff can get to know you and the patient. If you can afford it, consider getting a suite, which will be more comfortable, and will give you more space to move about.

If there is an apartment hotel available in the area, you may consider staying there. You might be able to make meals, and stick to a routine that is closer to the one you are used to at home. Consider using room service if you think managing meals in the dining-room will be too difficult.

To ensure security, inform the front desk of the hotel and the doorman about your relative's illness, and ask them to stop your family member from leaving when unaccompanied by you.

If you are invited to stay at someone's home, you should think about how comfortable you will be about allowing them to see your family member's problems first hand. You should also find out whether you are the only guests. If not, perhaps a small hotel would provide more quiet and privacy for you and the Alzheimer patient.

However, if you will feel comfortable staying with your hosts, and you will be able to establish routine in the household, you may find staying there preferable if the other people want to share the caregiving chores. If you are going for a social event such as a wedding, and have been invited to stay at the home of the guest of honour or a close relative such as the parents of the bride, there will probably be more excitement and commotion than an Alzheimer patient can comfortably handle.

In making your choice, your comfort and that of the patient should be the first consideration.

VACATIONS

When I found out Joe had Alzheimer Disease I assumed we'd never take another vacation together. But about six months later, we went with some friends to a Caribbean island for a week. We rented a two-bedroom apartment on the beach, and mostly just hung around, reading, walking on the beach, and just sitting. It took some ingenuity to keep Joe occupied, but we managed, and I was surprised how well it went. Having a kitchen in the apartment made it a lot easier. Unfortunately, Joe's condition got worse, and we couldn't go away together again.

Vacations are a special form of travel. In the early stages of your family member's disease, you can continue to take a family vacation, though it may be different from the kind you were used to.

A vacation that involves travelling to a number of different places or staying in a large, busy city can be difficult for a person with Alzheimer Disease. The city will probably give him or her more stimulation than he or she can handle, and travelling around is likely to be disorienting. A trip to a single destination where you can stay for the duration of the vacation is likely to be the most restful for you and the most satisfying for your family member. If there is a destination that you have always enjoyed and have been to often, you will already know your way around and this will make it easier for you to relax. Wherever you are, try to create a home-like environment and establish a daily routine.

If the Alzheimer patient is not used to sitting around all day, choose a place that can provide some diversions—a walk into town, strolling on the beach, looking in shops. If the person has never liked warm climates in the past, don't try a holiday in the South now.

You might want to take your holiday with friends. They can help you with the care of your family member and provide you with pleasurable diversions. Furthermore, you will probably feel more secure to have friends available as a back-up in case of emergency. Discuss the trip with your friends before you go and make sure that you are all clear about your expectations of each other during the trip.

As the Alzheimer patient's condition deteriorates, taking a vacation will become more difficult for both of you. The patient will become more dependent on the familiar surroundings, and will have difficulty adjusting to a new environment. Nevertheless, you may feel the need for a vacation from caregiving, and even the need to get away from your daily surroundings. In that case, check to see whether institutional respite-care is available.

SOCIAL EVENTS

You might be invited to a special social event such as a wedding, an anniversary party or birthday, or similar social occasion.

Deciding whether or not to accept the invitation involves several factors, and possibly some trade-offs. You will have to weigh the importance of the event to you, whether you think you will be able to enjoy yourself, the effect on yourself if you do not go, and how much trouble it will be to go. After all, the purpose of these events is to celebrate and have a good time. You must deal with the reality of the situation–how your family member will manage at the event–and you must also juggle your own feelings about guilt and fun.

Of course, you have several options. You may decide that both you and the patient will attend; that neither of you will go; or that you will go by yourself.

"It was my best friend's 40th anniversary. We've been friends since high school and it was important to me to be there. I told her Joe and I would come. But the day of the event, Joe was having a bad day. I called my daughter to stay with him, and went alone."

"Good for you. I could never have done that because I would have felt too guilty to leave my husband."

"I took Murray when he was having a bad day, and I was so busy worrying about him, I didn't enjoy myself. I wish I had left him home."

If you go alone, the guilt you may have to struggle with can take many forms. One is, of course, the guilt you feel about leaving your family member and going out. Your guilt may be stronger if you think the person could manage and you decided you would prefer to go by yourself, or if you are leaving your family member at home to spare yourself embarrassment.

The reverse side is the possibility of feeling badly that by not attending, you are disappointing those who have invited you to share a special occasion. The strength of this concern will probably vary with the importance of the event and how close you are to the people who invited you.

Among the realistic factors to consider is the nature of the event itself. Unstructured cocktail parties and receptions are probably the most difficult kind of social event for anybody to handle, and especially so for people with Alzheimer Disease.

The type of person your family member is also needs to be considered. If the person never enjoyed social events in the past, he or she probably won't enjoy them now either.

Another factor to consider is whether there is someone who can accompany you and the patient to the event. You could ask a live-in caregiver, a paid respite-worker, another family member or someone who helps you during the day and whom you trust. Be sure to confirm this arrangement with the hosts of the event.

It may make your decision easier if you plan to have the patient attend only a part of the event. However, some families have been surprised at how well an Alzheimer patient adapted to a large social function. The person's intellectual deficits did not seem to be a problem since the social skills were so well ingrained. This is not to say that the person was responsive to everyone, but the large numbers of people allowed the patient to use daily rituals to get by. The patient could smile and put a hand out to shake hands even if he or she didn't remember who was being introduced. The patient was able to say, "Hello, how are you?" to anyone who came along.

If you are invited to many social events in a short period of time, which often happens around Christmas, you will need to decide how many and which ones the Alzheimer patient can manage. Smaller events may be preferable, and those that will be attended by people well known to your family member.

When you decide to attend social events on your own, there is no reason to feel guilty. However, you will need to plan for someone to look after the patient while you are out. This is really the same as any other situation in which you need respite-care, and it would be advisable to use the same resources you usually do, be they family, friends or a paid respite-worker.

Before you go, you may want to think about what you will say to other people at the party when they ask about the patient. You do not need to go into great detail to everyone, but it is best to be open about the illness.

To those who know the situation, you need only say that you decided that it was best not to bring the patient. To those who don't know about your relative's illness, you need only say that he or she isn't well and couldn't attend. You can, of course, tell them what the illness is, but you should not feel obliged to do so.

If you decide both you and the Alzheimer patient will attend a party, you have to prepare the person. While you will probably want to tell the person ahead of time, he or she may not remember.

Even though you may be excited about going, try to remain relaxed to prevent your family member from becoming too agitated. The patient may not understand why you are excited, but will sense any extra expectations you place on him or her.

It is important to plan in advance. Decide what you will wear and what your family member will wear long enough ahead so you can have the clothing ready. This will prevent last minute panic, problematic before any big event, but especially so when your family member is easily disturbed.

Be sure that your family member is dressed appropriately, but comfortably. If the event requires formal wear, choose a dark suit for a man, and a nice street length dress for a woman. Avoid buying new clothes just for one occasion.

You may need to change the family routine to accommodate a special event. For example, it may be necessary to adjust mealtimes, so that your family member does not go too long without food. If you usually eat at 6:00, but dinner at a wedding won't be served until 8:00, give the person a snack before you leave. You may even want to carry some crackers or carrot strips with you.

You may also need to adjust the time that regular medication is given, especially if this medication helps the person relax. For example, you may need to give the patient half a pill before the event, instead of the whole pill before he or she goes to sleep. It would be a good idea to check with your family physician about how best to do this.

If possible, be responsible for your own transportation rather than relying on someone else, even if it means taking a taxi, because you can control when you leave. If another person is with you, he or she could go home with the patient and you could stay as long as you wish.

EATING IN RESTAURANTS

If you have always enjoyed eating out together, you do not have to stop with the onset of Alzheimer Disease. There are ways to adapt and modify the activity so that it is still pleasurable.

Some planning should go into choosing the restaurant. What were formerly your favourite restaurants may not be suitable now. Formal restaurants with a subdued atmosphere will not tolerate unusual behaviour as easily as a less formal family restaurant. However, bistros or cafés with loud music, or restaurants that are extremely noisy may be upsetting to an Alzheimer patient. Fast food chains have the advantage of fast service, allowing for anonymity, limited choice, and no necessity to deal with a waitress or waiting for a bill.

If you are in a family restaurant, try to choose a booth against a wall as opposed to a table in the middle of the room to reduce distractions. Instead of giving your relative a menu, give him or her limited choices if he or she can deal with it; or offer individual options until there is one that he or she accepts (would you like chicken? would you like fish?). If the person cannot handle making choices, you should do the ordering.

> I ordered an egg sandwich for my husband. The waitress turned to him and asked if he wanted it plain or toasted.

Even if the person has difficulty eating, he or she can likely handle finger foods in a restaurant. Chicken wings, vegetable sticks, hamburgers, hot dogs, and sandwiches are all easy to eat and acceptable. Make sure that the person is wearing clothes that are easily cleaned so that spills and messes will not be a serious problem. Try asking for the bill as soon as you order so that you can leave in a hurry if you have to.

CAREGIVING FROM A DISTANCE

> In a funny way, I'm the primary caregiver for my Uncle Pete, even though he lives about seven hundred miles from me. He lives alone and he never married. It's taken great planning and ingenuity on my part to be able to keep him at home as long as I have. I've really had to make maximum use of community resources, but so far it's working fine.

You may have responsibility for a relative who has Alzheimer Disease and lives alone in another community. Although you cannot be there on a daily basis to monitor what is happening, there are steps you can take to arrange for appropriate care at the person's home.

The key to making this work is to have a case manager in the patient's community. A case manager is a person who takes primary responsibility for co-ordinating all the services a patient will need. It is the case manager who contacts agencies, arranges for them to provide the needed services, and monitors the quality and reliability of the services. A case manager may be a social worker, a nurse, an occupational therapist or some other member of the helping professions.

A lot of the initial organizing and planning can be done from your home with long distance phone calls. However, at some point you will want to make a personal visit to be sure the organization of the care is working. You may also need to be physically present to make some of the arrangements.

Use the social agencies as resources in the community where the patient lives. You can also make contacts by getting names from the patient's doctor. If the patient lives in the United States contact the Alzheimer Disease and Related Disorders Association. If you have difficulty finding an association in your relative's community, contact the head office at 70 E. Lake St., Chicago, Illinois for the chapter nearest your relative's home.

I contacted the Family Service Association who visited Uncle Pete, did an assessment and told me I should come to see him. I could only get four days off from work, so before I went, I organized the visit. I arranged for a doctor to come to the house to do an assessment while I was there, and I got the name of a lawyer from the Family Service Association. I made an appointment to see the lawyer to discuss guardianship for my relative. I also found out which bank he used and contacted the manager to arrange an appointment to discuss on-going arrangements for paying Uncle Pete's bills. But the most important thing was to have a chance to meet the social worker who's doing case management for my uncle. After all, she's the person I depend on most, and I needed to be sure I had hired the right person. She goes to visit Uncle Pete once a week, and calls me once a month.

HOSPITALIZATION FOR OTHER REASONS

If a serious medical condition develops, it may be necessary to hospitalize an Alzheimer patient for other reasons. However, this should be avoided if at all possible, since the peculiar routine of hospitals can be disorienting to even the most focused individual. If surgery is needed, find out if the procedure can be done in a day surgery unit.

Contrary to what one might expect, most hospital personnel are relatively uninformed about the nature of Alzheimer Disease and how to deal with it. Hence, you will need to serve as advocate and interpreter for the patient and explain his or her needs and behaviour to hospital staff. You will also have to explain hospital procedures to your family member.

Some members of the hospital staff will have stereotyped images of Alzheimer patients and will assume your family member fits that stereotype. That image often includes an assumption that the person is incontinent, violent, or inclined to wander. If your family member is not incontinent, make sure the staff know that. You will need to emphasize to them the importance of responding quickly when the patient indicates a need to use the toilet or a bedpan.

Try not to let the hospital staff restrain the patient. This is only likely to increase agitation, and may result in injury. If necessary, try to get someone to stay with the patient as a way of countering the perceived need for restraints. Since you may need this care on a twenty-four hour basis, consider hiring someone since you will need some time away. If your family member does not need much professional nursing care, you may be able to use an aide or companion to stay with the person. If there is a paid caregiver at your house, perhaps he or she could provide care for your family member while he or she is in the hospital. It will be reassuring to the person to have someone familiar in the room.

Make sure hospital staff understand that they cannot rely on the patient to answer questions, nor can they rely on the accuracy of the answers if he or she does respond. You must supply the patient's history (those written records, including the drug records, will be helpful here). You should, if possible, be present when the person is examined, so you can help keep him or her calm and explain what is being done. You can also explain your family member's reactions and responses to those doing the examination.

Try to arrange for the patient to have a private room. This will be less disorienting than having a stranger in the next bed, and the Alzheimer patient could be disturbing to another patient.

If your family member is in for a short stay, you may wish to arrange to stay overnight, too. Many hospitals will permit you to put a cot in the room at night. If the patient doesn't have a private room, perhaps you could stay in a visitors' room on the same ward.

If there is an object or picture that is comforting and familiar to the patient, and it is easy to carry around, take it with you to the hospital for him or her. If your family member is not on a restricted diet, also bring favourite foods.

Should anesthesia be necessary, you should be with your family member when he or she wakes up to assist the person's orientation. Because anesthesia can be disorienting in the best of circumstances, you may expect the person to be more disoriented than usual following these procedures.

If you can't avoid a hospital stay, at least try to keep it as short as possible. Perhaps there is a long-term care facility near you with infirmary beds for people with Alzheimer Disease. That may be a good place for your family member to recover. Or, if you can afford it, take the person home and hire a special nurse.

If your family member has to go to the Emergency Room, inform Emergency Room staff that he or she has Alzheimer Disease as soon as you arrive. See if there is a separate room where you can wait, away from the hustle and bustle of the main Emergency waiting room. Be sure to monitor medication anyone may give your family member, since some drugs can affect the person's behaviour.

If you have a long wait in an Emergency Room, make use of the support network you have. Call someone–a friend, another family member–to come and wait with you. It's stressful enough to wait in an Emergency Room without the added stress of having to be with someone who has Alzheimer Disease. Besides, if you need to leave the waiting room to talk to the doctor, use the washroom, or even get a cup of coffee, you will want someone who knows the patient to stay with him or her.

WHEN THE CAREGIVER HAS
AN EMERGENCY

There may be times when you suddenly discover that you cannot take care of the Alzheimer patient. Perhaps you have had a fall and must go to the hospital for an x-ray, or you have a flu, or you have a serious and sudden illness that requires hospitalization.

If you are experiencing an emergency, be sure to look after your own needs as well as those of your family member, and in this case, your own needs may well take precedence over those of the Alzheimer patient. If you have a heart attack, you must get medical help right away, even if it means taking the Alzheimer patient in the ambulance with you. You can, however, reduce the impact of this kind of problem by planning ahead, so that in an emergency you know what you will do.

During an emergency is the time to use your network. Choose one person in your support network as the first one you will contact in an emergency. This person's job will be to come right away, and help you through the first stages, until you can make another arrangement. Ideally, it will be someone who lives close by, and who is able to come immediately. You may not have too many choices, but try to choose someone with a flexible job and life-style, who can drop work at a moment's notice.

If you are unable to care for your family member for a long period of time, you will need to make some alternate arrangements. None of them are likely to be ideal, but you'll have to make some plans so that the patient has care while you are unavailable.

One option is to contact places in your community that provide institutional respite. Alternatively, you can contact your home-care agency for a live-in homemaker to stay with the patient until you are well again. A third possibility is to contact a commercial agency for a live-in homemaker. You may need to use a combination of these solutions, or there may be someone in your family or support network who can move in and provide care alone or in conjunction with one of the other alternatives.

While no one likes to think about emergencies, you would be wise to plan for an emergency before it happens. Once you have identified the options for longer-term care, talk to your emergency back-up person about what the options are, what your preferences are, and who to contact to make arrangements when you can't. If you have records of important information such as your family member's medication schedule, his likes and dislikes, and his daily routine, be sure your emergency helper knows where you keep this information. Remember, you may not be able to communicate with the people who are caring for your family member in an emergency.

MOVING HOUSE

There are many reasons why a household may need to move. Your house may be too large, or may have too many stairs. Perhaps you want to live near other family members who could help you with emotional support and respite-care. There may be financial reasons that motivate your move.

Despite all of these very valid reasons, we do not recommend moving. It will be very stressful for you, and the physical changes will be extremely disorienting for an Alzheimer patient. At the best of times, moving means boxes on the floor, and your life is in chaos. For a person with Alzheimer Disease, moving is even more difficult.

Nevertheless, if you *must* move, do some careful planning. If you anticipate that you will not be able to continue with your current doctor, inform your family doctor of the move and ask for referrals in your new neighbourhood. Check with your local Alzheimer chapter for the community services available. Visit the neighbourhood before the move to familiarize yourself with shopping and services so that you will know what to expect.

Make sure that someone will take care of the Alzheimer patient out of the house the day of the move. Pack the patient's most familiar objects last to minimize the disorienting effect of moving. If possible, have the person participate in the move by packing some of his or her own things.

Moving is a time when you need your friends' help. It will be more comfortable and less disorienting if familiar people are present in the new house or apartment. Friends could help you unpack or spend time with the patient while you are unpacking and organizing.

After you have moved to your new residence, the Alzheimer patient will likely be upset. Nothing will look the same. To alleviate the person's anxiety, unpack things that are familiar and put them in place right away. Now is not the time to redecorate or to try out new furnishings. Try to keep the new place as close to the appearance of the old as possible. For example, hang the same pictures and don't put the living-room chair in the bedroom.

During the first few days after you move, try to stay with the patient as much as possible to reassure him or her that you are still there. Try to engage the person in the daily routine so that he or she will become familiar with the new surroundings.

Make sure that all the safety issues that you took care of in your previous residence have been covered.

Just as you did before, begin to develop your community network. You may already know someone in your new neighbourhood. Start there and use the person to help you build a new support network. Meet your new neighbours and get to know them so that you can be comfortable explaining your relative's situation. Have them alert you if they see the patient outside alone.

If you move to an apartment, you should introduce your family member to the staff in your building. Explain that the person has Alzheimer Disease, and what that means. Then they can be alert to potential problems. If the building has a doorman, be sure he is aware of the possibility that the patient may wander.

AUTOPSY

An autopsy is an examination of a person's body after death, usually for the purpose of determining the cause of death. In the case of Alzheimer Disease, it is the only certain way of diagnosing the disease. This is why you may be approached by your attending physician for permission to allow an autopsy of your family member's body.

Because autopsies have a great deal to contribute to our understanding of Alzheimer Disease and its possible causes, we encourage you to agree to an autopsy request, unless it is against your religious beliefs. The person's body will not be disfigured as a result of the autopsy.

A release is required to give the doctor permission to perform an autopsy. It is often possible to sign this form before a person's death, so you will not have to be concerned about it at a more difficult time. When the patient dies, you will only need to confirm that you have given permission for an autopsy.

There is some urgency to performing the autopsy immediately after death, since the brain contains enzymes that destroy many of the clues to the cause of Alzheimer Disease. If you are prepared to grant permission for an autopsy, you should let the doctor know in advance. You should also be sure that whoever is looking after the patient in the terminal stages is also aware of your decision, so that proper arrangements can be made quickly after the patient's death. If you are interested in the results of the autopsy for yourself, inform the doctor.

FURTHER READING

Safford, Florence. *Caring for the Mentally Impaired Elderly: A Family Guide*. New York: Henry Holt and Company, 1987.

Shroyer, Jo Ann L. and Hutton, J. Thomas. "Optimal Living Environments For Alzheimer Patients," in Dippel, Raye Lynne and Hutton, Thomas J. (Eds), *Caring for the Alzheimer Patient: A Practical Guide*. Buffalo, New York: Prometheus Books, 1988.

12

COMMUNICATION

❦

C hanges in communication skills are among the first and most frequently noted signs of Alzheimer Disease.
Patients of the disease have two kinds of communication problems. Difficulty with expressing oneself is called an *expressive* communication problem. This includes difficulty in remembering a word, a name, or a phrase and it is among the most common early signs of Alzheimer Disease. Alzheimer patients may also have difficulty with *receptive* communication, that is, with understanding information given to him or her.

This chapter offers insights into communication problems Alzheimer patients have, and suggests some practical ways of compensating for them.

It is often easier to notice when people have problems expressing themselves than to notice when they are having problems understanding what we are saying. Consequently, we often tend to focus on the expressive problems of people with Alzheimer Disease, particularly in the early phases when communication problems first develop. Nevertheless, even at this early stage, you should be alert to the possibility that your family member is having difficulty with receptive as well as expressive communication.

EXPRESSIVE COMMUNICATION

The earliest problems with expressive communication have to do with the words for objects, or the names of people and places. An Alzheimer patient may have difficulty remembering–and therefore, using—words, especially nouns. Because this initially involves a specific word, a person may be fairly adept at overcoming the problem by describing the object for which she or he has forgotten the name.

When Mrs. Green wanted to listen to the radio, but couldn't remember the word, she asked where "the box that the music and voices come out of" was.

Later on, Alzheimer patients often substitute a related word for the word they cannot remember: sister for daughter, spoon for fork, blouse for skirt.

When an Alzheimer patient has difficulty finding the correct word, you should supply it, though in a tactful way that helps to preserve a person's dignity. Do not simply fill in the word. Rather, you can use a sentence that includes the correct word the person is groping for, such as:

Mr. Johnson (while holding his coffee cup): Please pass me the . . . the . . . the . . .
Mrs. Johnson: Here is the milk for your coffee.

Another approach is to suggest the correct word as one of two alternatives, even if you know which one the person really means.

Mr. Black (holding a knife, with toast on his breakfast plate): I'd like some . . . some . . .
Mrs. Black: Would you like butter or jam for your toast?

As the disease progresses and the patient's problems expand from difficulty with individual words to difficulty with ideas, there will be a noticeable change in the quality of the person's oral expression. He or she will talk around the topic of conversation, without directly addressing a subject. This is called circumlocution, literally "to talk around."

When I asked my mother what she had for dinner tonight, she replied, "Oh, your father is a wonderful cook."

Sometimes the circumlocutions can become a great deal more elaborated, as the patient strings together words and phrases that on first hearing seem to relate to the topic and to make great sense; in fact, sometimes they may even sound reasonably profound. However, careful listening will reveal that what is being said does not really answer the question or make a great deal of sense, and often consists of a series of ritualistic expressions that the person has used often in the past.

"Harry, how do you like the day centre?"

"It's okay. It's sort of interesting, you know."

"What do you do at the day centre?"

"Well, you know, it's a kind of interesting concept. It's a new program, you know, so the concept is evolving; they haven't actually really fully established the concept, but it's evolving and it's quite an interesting one."

"When you are there, how do you spend your day?"

"Well, as I said, it's not too clearly established. They are trying to let the concept evolve, and they haven't clearly established it yet, but I think it will be quite an interesting concept when they finally have it sorted out, and have let it evolve to what it could be."

When a person starts talking this way, it is important that you listen to the sense of what is being said, rather than to the specifics. If you really need to understand what the person is trying to say, listen to the generalities and then ask specific questions that he or she can answer relatively easily. Questions that can be answered with a "yes" or "no" are particularly useful in obtaining specific information.

The ability to sound intelligent can be particularly deceptive because of the high level of social skills that people with Alzheimer Disease often retain well into the course of the illness. And if a person is having a "good day," he or she may succeed in fooling even an aware and astute observer for a short period of time.

A colleague and I went to visit a unit for people with Alzheimer Disease in a long-term-care setting. As we entered the unit, a handsome and well groomed older man greeted us at the door and asked if he could help us. When I told him I was looking for Joanne [the head nurse on the unit] he politely informed me that she was in a meeting, that he thought the meeting would last about another ten minutes, and that he was sure she would be happy to meet with me when the meeting was over. In the meantime, he suggested, I could wait for her near the nurses' station. When I replied that we would like to walk around the unit and look at how it was decorated, he assured me that would be fine, and offered to let Joanne know that someone was here to see her as soon as her meeting was over. Because he was so very helpful and articulate, and because I knew this setting was very careful about who it admitted to its special unit, I suggested to my colleague that this man must be a volunteer on the unit.

While I was touring around the unit, I met the head nurse and spoke to her about the matter I had come to discuss. As I was leaving the unit, the same man was at the door. When I thanked him for his help and said I had met with Joanne, he looked at me blankly for a moment, then said that his mother was coming to visit him later and she and he would be leaving on a vacation for Europe in a few hours. This was totally out of context, and I realized that this well-spoken man was actually a resident of the unit who was now out of touch with reality.

RECEPTIVE COMMUNICATION

Problems with receptive communication may be harder to identify. However, if an Alzheimer patient does not respond when you speak to him or her, you should consider the probability that he or she is having difficulty understanding what you are saying. In the early stages this is less noticeable, but it does occur. It is not clear whether early difficulties in receptive communication result from forgetting the meaning of a word or from an inability to comprehend what is said.

When an Alzheimer patient shows difficulties with receptive communication, it could also be because of a hearing problem. Remember that your family member will experience other age-related changes along with Alzheimer Disease.

If the person has been wearing a hearing-aid, you should check that he or she is still using it and that it works well. Since the patient will no longer be able to look after the aid himself, you should learn how to do it. A clinical audiologist can teach you how to clean it, how to check the batteries, and how to change them when necessary. Wearing a hearing-aid that is not working is like putting your finger in your ear because the ear mould blocks the entry of sound to the ear.

If the patient has not had his or her hearing checked in the last two years, you should arrange for this to be done. Do not be put off by the fact that he has Alzheimer Disease. A qualified audiologist can carry out a hearing assessment even if a person has difficulty understanding and responding to instructions. To find a qualified audiologist, contact the audiology or speech pathology department of your local hospital. If the hospital doesn't have either of these departments, call the local branch of the Canadian Hearing Society or ask a doctor who specializes in ear, nose, and throat problems to give you the name of a qualified audiologist.

If the audiologist discovers that an Alzheimer patient has a hearing loss, it is probably not worth getting a hearing aid. Unlike glasses, the person would have to learn to use the aid and this is a skill that is probably beyond his or her abilities. However, there are other things you can do to help compensate for the hearing loss.

1. Make sure the person can see you when you are talking to him or her. Stand where the person can see your face easily when you are talking. If the person uses glasses, make sure he or she wears them when needing to hear. There is truth to the old joke, "Just a minute till I put my glasses on. I can't hear you."

2. You can purchase mechanical devices that amplify the voice of the speaker in much the same way as a microphone. Because these are used by the caregiver instead of the person with Alzheimer Disease, they may be useful for dealing with an Alzheimer patient who also has a hearing loss.

    A sophisticated version of this concept involves talking into earphones worn by the patient. Not only will this magnify your voice, but may have the added advantage of helping the person focus on what you are saying. However, some people have found that an Alzheimer patient becomes agitated when wearing earphones. This clearly negates other benefits obtained from this approach.

    Talk to a qualified audiologist before deciding to use mechanical devices.

As the Alzheimer patient's abilities deteriorate, he or she will find it progressively more difficult to understand spoken language. If you want to try to imagine what this is like, listen to a television or radio program in a language you don't understand. As you become bored and restless, you will perhaps come to understand your relative's own reaction to these media, and why he or she fiddles with the dials (perhaps in an attempt to tune in to the station better).

For the same reasons, some patients, at a certain stage, may stop listening to music, since music is a language with a structure that requires concentration if one is to really understand it. (There is a difference between actively listening to music and using it as background sound. Many people report that Alzheimer patients enjoy listening to music that is familiar to them and is of the easy listening variety.)

Some caregivers have found that a patient is better able to listen to music through earphones, since this reduces distraction and allows for more concentration on the music. However, some Alzheimer patients do not feel comfortable wearing earphones.

NON-VERBAL COMMUNICATION

Only some of the things we communicate are communicated with words. The rest of our messages use non-verbal forms of communication—our tone of voice, our facial expressions, gestures, hands, posture, and pictures. In fact, non-verbal methods may account for more than half of what we communicate.

As a patient's ability to use and understand oral communication deteriorates, you will have to increase your reliance on non-verbal communication. When the patient can no longer use words to convey feelings or needs, pay attention to what he or she is trying to tell you through gestures, posture, and facial expressions.

Most people with Alzheimer Disease can understand non-verbal communication even after they can no longer understand verbal communication. In fact, in the final stages of the disease, Alzheimer patients lose the ability to express and understand speech, but remain responsive to touch and tone of voice. You can use this responsiveness to non-verbal communication to advantage in communicating with the patient.

TIPS FOR COMMUNICATING WITH
A PATIENT

- Approach the patient slowly and from the front. If you rush at the person, he or she may think you are about to attack.

- Use a friendly tone of voice.

- Because your family member may have difficulty making sense of too much information, keep background stimulation (a television, radio or stereo, or other conversations) to a minimum when you are trying to talk to him or her.

- Be sure you have the patient's attention before you start to speak. Touch him or her gently on the arm or hand, call the person by name, and stand where he or she can see your face while you talk.

- Maintain eye contact throughout the conversation, and use the person's name repeatedly while you are talking.

- Speak slowly and clearly so the person can understand you. Use short sentences and simple words.

- Be patient. It may take a while for the person to understand what you are saying or asking. Don't rush. Present one idea at a time, and repeat it until you are sure your family member has grasped it.

- When asking questions, try to frame them so the person can give a simple and specific response. Instead of asking "What would you like to do now?" offer a specific option to which the person can say "yes" or "no" ("Would you like to watch some television?"). Don't ask a second question until the first one has been answered.

- Don't ask questions or present options unless you really mean it. If you ask the patient if he or she would like to watch television and the response is "no" don't decide you'd like to watch it anyway and turn it on.

- Because people with Alzheimer Disease have lost the ability for abstract thinking, they will often take what you say quite literally. Be very precise in your use of language and choose your words carefully. Be sure to say what you mean, and avoid using euphemisms.

   For example, if you want the person to use the toilet, say so. Using a euphemism such as "Would you like to wash your hands?" may lead him to say no, even if he really does need to use the toilet. Besides, you've also broken the rule about not giving someone a choice unless you really mean it.

My wife helped me make fruit salad in the kitchen. When it was all mixed up in the serving bowl, I told her to put the fruit salad on the tray, so I could take it to the table. She picked up the bowl, and poured the fruit salad directly on to the tray. She really had put the fruit salad on the tray.

- Use non-verbal cues such as gestures to reinforce what you are saying. If you want to ask the patient if he or she would like to watch television, point to the person and to the television while you are saying these words.

- Use symbols, pictures, and objects to help communicate. If the person cannot remember which cabinet has the cups and saucers, put a picture of them on the door. Involve the patient in selecting the picture, so you can be sure he or she will recognize it later.

Use the skull and crossbones symbols to indicate things that are dangerous. It is a commonly accepted symbol for marking poisons, but can be used to mark other places where dangerous things are stored–sharp knives, medicine, even knobs on the stove.

If a patient reacts badly when you say it is time to take a bath, it may be because he or she has forgotten what that means. Handing him or her soap and a towel, objects associated with taking a bath, might clarify the message.

- Use your facial expression, your tone of voice and your posture to convey your feelings. People with Alzheimer Disease are extremely sensitive to social cues, and while they may not understand the specific meaning from the words you are using, they will understand the general sense of your feelings from these non-verbal cues.

Be sure your verbal and non-verbal cues are consistent with each other; inconsistency will only add to a patient's confusion and difficulty in understanding communication. Don't tell your family member you're not angry if the non-verbal cues say you are. Don't be sarcastic towards the person; sarcasm and irony are lost on people with Alzheimer Disease.

WRITING MESSAGES

You may be surprised to discover that the Alzheimer patient is still able to read and understand even after he or she has difficulty comprehending oral speech. For a long time it was believed that people with Alzheimer Disease could read words, but could not understand what they meant. However, recent research indicates that under certain specific conditions, Alzheimer patients can read and understand what they are reading even though they no longer understand spoken language.[1]

This finding has important implications, because it means you can extend the period when you are able to communicate with an Alzheimer patient by writing notes. If you print simple notes in large clear letters, and if the person reads these notes aloud several times

[1]Adapted from Irene Campbell-Taylor and M. Behrmann, "Semantics and Reading Ability in Alzheimer Disease," *Brain and Language* (in press), 1989.

over until you can tell from the reading that he or she understands, you can use this method to communicate.

This is a somewhat slow and tedious process, so you will probably want to reserve this method of communicating for important things. For example, if you suspect that the person has a pain, you might print a note that says, "Do I have a pain?" (Notice the use of "I" rather than "you" in the note. If the note had read "Do you have a pain?" the person might find this confusing, on the grounds that he or she doesn't know how you feel.) If the patient read the note aloud several times until you could tell he or she understood, and then the person answered you by saying that he or she did have a pain, you could then write a series of successive notes about possible locations of the pain. (Is the pain in my head? Is the pain in my stomach?)

While this finding about an Alzheimer patient's reading comprehension is useful, this approach will work only under the following conditions:

Your relative must read the note aloud.
The person must read it as often as necessary until you are sure he or she really does understand—that is, until the person answers the question in the note.

Because this approach works only under these specific conditions, you must be present when the patient is reading the note.

This is quite a different situation from leaving your family member a note as a reminder to do something if you have left him or her alone for an extended period. For example, in the early stages of your family member's disease, you may feel comfortable about leaving him or her alone for the day, but you may want to leave a note to remind the person to have lunch. The difficulty with this is that even though the person may still be able to read, he or she may not remember to read the note. It is preferable for someone—yourself, a friend, or another member of the family—to phone the patient at the appropriate time with a reminder.

FURTHER READING

Ostuni, Elizabeth & Santo Pietro, Mary Jo. *Getting Through: Communicating When Someone You Care For Has Alzheimer's Disease.* Princeton, New Jersey: Speech Bin, 1986.

13
THE ENVIRONMENT

❦

In previous chapters we have discussed a variety of problems relating to Alzheimer Disease that are difficult to control. However, the issue of environmental safety is one aspect of care that you can control. By modifying your home to improve the health and safety of your family member, you will allow all members of the household to function more comfortably. This chapter will focus on environmental changes that are inexpensive and easy to implement and will make your home environment a safe place for you and your family member.

We have suggested that all aspects of care for your family member should be structured. Since the environment is an aspect of the care you provide, your family member will function better in an ordered environment. As you minimize choice in other matters, you should also minimize choice with respect to the environment. The way you deal with the environment will change as your relative's disease progresses. You will need to adapt the environment so that it provides progressively less stimulation.

Just as a structured and ordered day is essential, so is a structured and ordered environment. The environment is the source of aural (sounds) and visual stimulation. When an Alzheimer patient needs to focus on a specific activity to complete a task, too much stimulation can be distracting and frustrating. If a patient is trying to wash, and hand soap, liquid soap, and several small guest soaps arranged in a basket are available, he or she will find it confusing to make a choice. This does not mean that you cannot keep things you like around the house. However, we do suggest that you keep only a few such things on display to avoid more stimulation than your family member can process.

While environmental modifications will be necessary in order to make the environment safe and to help your family member function at a higher level, try not to make changes unless they are necessary, since changes in the environment are difficult for a patient to handle. Do not rearrange furniture unless there is a good reason and do not move utensils, clothing, or other objects that your family member may still be able to use independently. You may think you should move the plates to a place where he or she will find them more easily, but it is more likely that the change will cause confusion and make the plates harder, rather than easier, for your family member to find.

Try to maintain existing routines that relate to the environment so that your family member will associate a particular activity with a particular location. For example, if you have always eaten dinner in the dining room, try not to eat dinner in the kitchen, even if that would be easier. You may find that the kitchen is easier to clean but that it is harder to get your family member to sit down and eat there.

The appearance of the environment can provide an Alzheimer patient with a cue about the kinds of behaviours that are expected in a particular space. A bedroom obviously looks different from a dining room – the bed tells your family member that this is a place to sleep.

There are other ways to use the environment to help your family member deal with memory loss and disorientation. Specific examples that you can apply in the rooms in your own home are discussed below. (You can also refer to Chapter 10, which has a detailed section on wandering and suggestions of various modifications you could make to your home to make it safer.)

ADAPTING YOUR HOME ENVIRONMENT

KITCHEN

Adjust your stove so that the patient cannot use the burners or the oven when you are not there. If you have an electric stove, you may be able to install an extra switch that must be activated before the stove will work, or you may need to remove the knobs, the fuses, or the circuit breaker. If you have a gas stove, contact the gas company to see what can be done. Other dangers in the kitchen include sharp objects. Place knives and scissors where your family member cannot get to them.

When your family member can no longer remember where to put away the dinner plates and glasses, you can put pictures of these items on the cupboards where they belong.

When the Alzheimer patient has difficulty keeping track of time, a clock with large, easy-to-read numbers may help for a while. Similarly, a calendar with large numbers may help the person keep track of days and dates. You can use either the kind in which you tear off a page for each day, or you can use a picture calendar with one month on each page. If you use a picture calendar, cross off each day as it is completed. A calendar in which the pictures correspond to the month (as opposed to a whole year of cats and dogs) is best.

BATHROOM

Even small aspects of the environment can help to cue behaviours. Your family member may be more apt to remember to wash his hands if the soap and towel are easily visible. A further cue for your family member would be to paint the taps in the sink and the bathtub red and blue for hot and cold so that he or she will know which to use. This is also a good safety precaution to prevent your family member from being scalded by hot water.

There are many items in the bathroom that can be dangerous for a person with Alzheimer Disease. Lock away hairdryers, razors, and any cleaning supplies. Remember also that all medications must be kept locked securely. Another safety feature would be to provide handrails and grab bars for your relative. Watch for spills on the floor in the bathroom and keep it dry at all times.

LIVING AREAS AND OPEN SPACES

People with Alzheimer Disease often retain good long-term memory and enjoy reminiscing about the past. You can encourage this through the kinds of things you use to decorate your home. A grouping of family pictures from the past may prompt some conversation about the family. Small mementos from a trip or a gift for a special occasion, such as a wedding or anniversary present, may help you and your family member reminisce about those events. Even furniture, if it has some special associations from the past, can help a person remember.

Put away valuable items that your family member might break or throw out. Include knick-knacks, jewellery, and other valuables.

Remember that an Alzheimer patient may, in confusion, throw these items out, give them away, or hide them where they cannot be found. These items will also clutter an area and will therefore distract or confuse the Alzheimer patient. Make a list of where you have placed these valuables.

If your house is carpeted, make sure all the edges are well tacked down and that there are no bumps or ridges to trip over. Remove small scatter or throw rugs since it is easy to slip and fall on them, especially at night. Use nightlights throughout the house to help your family member find the way in the middle of the night.

Place gates at the top and bottom of stairs so that your family member cannot use them when you are not there. As physical abilities deteriorate, stairs can be a source of accidents. Reduce the temperature on the hot water heater so scalding will not be possible even if your family member only turns on the hot water. Keep the door to the basement locked. Have radiator covers made to protect your family member from burning himself or herself on any exposed pipes. Identify other heat-producing sources and cover them as well.

Remove locks from room doors so your family member cannot lock himself or herself in a room. If you have drawers with built-in locks or cabinet or closet doors with locks, make sure the patient cannot lock them unless you yourself have a key. You may want to remove the lock or you may want to permanently lock the item and keep the key in a safe place where your relative cannot find it.

WORKROOM

Lock up all products such as cleaning supplies, paints, solvents, insecticides, gasoline, and kerosene. Include in your list those items that would be dangerous for your family member to swallow and any products that might harm him or her or damage your home. Remember to carefully label these items before you lock them up in case an accident does occur. Lock up sharp tools: knives, scissors, paper cutters, saws, drills, garden tools and screwdrivers. Other household dangers include irons, lawnmowers, and any appliances that could turn into fire hazards.

AGE-RELATED VISUAL CHANGES

There are aspects of environmental design for all older adults that are particularly important for people with Alzheimer Disease. These relate to changes in vision that occur with age. These changes can result in problems that are particularly disorienting for people with

Alzheimer Disease who may have special difficulty interpreting what they are seeing.

Age-related changes in the structure of the eye cause older people to be particularly sensitive to glare. Not only does this pose a safety hazard, since the glare makes it difficult for them to see, but the glare can be frightening and disorienting. The reflection of light on highly polished floors, such as in the kitchen and bathroom, may cause confusing optical illusions to your family member. Since a floor does not have to be shiny to be clean, you can reduce glare by cleaning but not waxing it. Not only will you make life easier for your family member, but you will have less work, too.

If glare is coming in through the windows, use horizontal or vertical blinds, shades or curtains to reduce it when it causes a problem. You may also want to check the position of the television to ensure that glare from a window is not reflecting onto the screen.

Since people's vision deteriorates with age, the use of light-dark contrast helps them read the environment more easily. Note that what is being discussed here is contrast between lightness and darkness and not necessarily contrast between different colours. Contrast between lightness and darkness may be thought of in terms of the amount of "colour" in the colour.

Contrast can help us understand the environment better when it is used along edges of stairs or furniture. If a table and the floor beneath it are both dark brown, your family member may have difficulty seeing where the edge of the table is, particularly since people with Alzheimer Disease often have difficulty with depth perception.

It is also important to use contrast in dealing with small and detailed aspects of the environment. For example, providing contrast between a plate and the surface it sits on is a good idea. A white plate on a white tablecloth will be harder for your family member to see than the same white plate on a dark blue placemat.

One woman reported that her husband often had difficulty urinating into the toilet and often ended up messing the floor. She finally hit on the idea of painting the toilet seat and tried several different colours until she found that bright orange worked well. He had had difficulty making sense of the all-white bathroom.

Contrast is sometimes important in helping us find things. If you have ever laid an aspirin on a white counter while you went to fill the water glass and then couldn't find the aspirin when the glass was full, you will understand the concept. Towel bars that contrast with the wall and towels in a third colour will make it easier for your family member to wash and dry his or her own hands.

Because of difficulties with depth perception as a result of Alzheimer Disease and the normal aging problems such as astigmatism and a decrease in visual acuity, the use of contrast is an important factor in helping the elderly navigate the environment safely.

Now that you have an understanding of principles such as glare and contrast, it is now possible to discuss how older people perceive actual "colours." These suggestions can be helpful in situations where you need to know what will stand out for the patient or what he or she will probably not notice.

Because of the yellowing of the lens, many elderly have difficulty distinguishing between blue and green, which may appear grey. Pastel shades often appear "washed out" and very difficult to see. Dark colours, such as maroon, dark brown, navy, and black, often appear "muddy" to the older person and should be avoided all together if possible. Red, orange, and yellow are the easiest colours for older people to see but excessive use of these colours might be unpleasant.

We hope it is now clear that it is possible to control the environment and provide a safe and secure home for your family member. You will need to know your family member's limits and realize that he or she is unable to take responsibility for his or her own safety. Learn to watch for potential hazards so that you can prevent accidents before they happen.

14

LONG-TERM CARE

❦

D eciding when you can no longer care for the Alzheimer patient at home is one of the most difficult decisions you will have to make in the course of the illness. You want to care for your family member at home for as long as possible, and you may want to make it possible for her or him to die at home. However, you must face the possibility that in the late stages of the disease the patient will require more care than you can provide.

In this chapter, you will find help for thinking through the question of how long you can care for the person at home; how to plan for the eventuality of having to put your family member in a long-term care setting; the features you should be looking for in such a setting; and some suggestions for making the transition into the setting as easy as possible for you and your family member.

FACTORS TO CONSIDER

1. *"Caregiver burden"* Caregiver burden is a phrase that has been coined to describe the strain experienced by family members who are providing long-term care to elderly relatives. It will probably be the most important factor in deciding when to put a patient into a long-term care setting.

    Different individuals have different abilities to manage the stresses of caregiving, so not all people will use the same marker to determine when a patient should move to a long-term care setting. Many people move the patient when he or she has lost control of the bowels. For other people, the need to move the patient happens earlier in the course of the disease, and some people are able to care for the patient at home throughout the entire course of the disease.

In response to our comments that we were preparing a section on when to move your relative into long-term care, a family member who had already been through that experience replied, "It's really very simple. When you say, 'I bloody well can't take any more of this,' it's time!"

2. *Effects on Health* Caregiver burden may be a psychological matter, or it may be a physical one. If the demands of caring for your family member are causing you to neglect your own health–not eating right, forgetting to take medication, lack of sleep because of the patient's night wandering–you should consider finding an alternative setting. After all, if you become ill as a result of your caregiving, the well-being of you and your family member are jeopardized at the same time.

3. *Effect on Other Household Members* If there are people living in your household besides you and the person you are caring for, you may need to think about how the situation is affecting them. Young children will continue to require your care and attention, and even older children, however understanding they may be, require time with an attentive parent. In some cases, the effect of an Alzheimer patient on other members of the household may be indirect and subtle, but still intense.

One day I brought my nine-year-old daughter and her friend to our house to play after school. When the car stopped, my daughter jumped out and ran inside, saying, "I'd better just make sure everything's okay first." Her father had started to undress himself, and she wanted to make sure he was decent before her friend came in. That was when I realized it was time to start thinking about finding a nursing home for him.

4. *Quality of Life* Community resources, such as those described in Chapter 5, will help you keep your relative at home for a long time. However, as difficult as it may be for you to accept, there may come a point when the patient's quality of life would be as good or better in long-term care than in your home. Your family member may find it easier to live in a situation with other people like himself, where programs and activities are structured especially to meet the needs and abilities of Alzheimer patients, and where staff are specially trained to provide the kind of stimulation, care, and support that people with Alzheimer Disease require.

HANDLING YOUR GUILT

It is easy to say that you should not feel guilty about putting your family member into a long-term care setting–and you should not. But we also know that saying you shouldn't feel guilty and actually not feeling guilty are not the same thing, since guilt is an irrational feeling. However, there are ways to overcome your guilt feelings.

1. Try to focus on the facts rather than the feelings. Think about how long you have given care, and about how it has affected you, the person with Alzheimer Disease, and other members of your family. Also consider how the situation may change for the better for all concerned after your family member is no longer living at home.

2. Try not to be concerned about what other people may think. You know your needs and your family member's needs better than anybody else. It's easy for other people to judge your behaviour, even when they are not knowledgeable and are not directly affected by your decision. Their judgmental response is their problem, not yours.

3. Discuss your decision with other members of your family. If they feel you should continue to provide care at home, ask them how they are prepared to help you.

4. Remember that other people have also moved Alzheimer patients to long-term care settings when they could no longer give care at home. Discuss your decision with some of these people. Try to find a family support group and talk to other caregivers who have had the same experience. Discuss your guilt feeling with them, and find out how they handled guilt, and whether they still feel the same way.

5. Meet with a professional counsellor to discuss your options and your feelings about the different choices you have. If possible, find a counsellor who specializes in counselling the elderly and their families with problems of aging. You might find such a person through a local family services agency or a religiously based counselling agency; or perhaps your family doctor can refer you to someone. Some long-term care settings have staff who can counsel you, or you can call the association of professional social workers in your province to see if they have a list of social workers in your community who specialize in this work.

6. Make an informed decision. Determine what your specific options are before you make a firm decision. Find out what settings are available to care for your family member, and visit those you wish to consider seriously.

7. Move your family member to a long-term care setting on a trial basis, by taking advantage of a respite-care program in your community. See how your family member fares, and observe your own reactions as well. Note, however, that you must take your family member home after the respite-period you and the setting have agreed to. Respite-care should never be seen as a "back door" for admission to a long-term care setting.

   While your family member's initial reaction may not be as good as you would wish, you should also realize that it may take staff a while to learn about the person's particular special needs and behavioural quirks. The longer they care for him, the better the care is likely to become.

8. Remember that placing the patient in a long-term care setting does not mean you are abandoning him or her. While you will no longer be the primary caregiver, you can continue to provide as much care as you are capable of, and you can visit the person regularly.

PLANNING FOR PLACEMENT

Even though we all wish to put off difficult decisions for as long as possible, there are several reasons why it is important to begin to think about placing your family member in a long-term care setting long before the need actually exists.

1. Long-term care facilities often have long waiting lists. If you wait to make application until the need is acute, and then have to wait until space is available, you may find that you have passed the point where you can cope with the strain of caregiving.

2. It is often difficult to find an appropriate setting for a patient. Some settings will not accept people with Alzheimer Disease, and others may not provide the quality of care you want. Consequently, you should be able to take time to look carefully at the alternatives before you make application. Waiting until there is a crisis will cause difficulty in checking out different settings.

If you have to rush to find a facility and move your family member to a setting that is inappropriate because you are in crisis, you run the risk of feeling guilty twice—once for placing the patient, and once again for placing him or her inappropriately.

In highlighting the importance of planning ahead, we are merely urging you to start thinking about the possibility that you may need to find a long-term care setting for your relative. Once you have overcome that hurdle, you should begin to look for settings where you would feel comfortable having your family member live. This does not mean that you should make application immediately. In fact, in many cases this is to be avoided, since it could result in the patient moving before it is necessary.

If a place became available and you turned it down because you are still able to care for your family member at home, you may find the patient's name at the bottom of the waiting list again. Hence, the timing for making application is a delicate issue, and you may wish to get professional advice on how to deal with this problem. People you could consult include a social worker who is knowledgeable about aging; the administrator of a setting where you are considering applying; your family doctor; a member of the team that initially assessed the patient; or someone at the central placement service, if there is one in your community.

HOW TO FIND A GOOD SETTING

In deciding which setting or settings (you can usually apply to more than one) you will apply to, the first step is to make a list of those you want to consider. When you have that list, you should plan to visit each one to evaluate it. Here are some ways to develop your list.

1. Some communities have a central assessment and placement service that coordinates admission to long-term care facilities. If your community has such a service, you will need to work through them so you should contact them first.

   Most central placement services allow their clients some choice in the facilities for which their family member will be considered. Thus, it is important that you meet with someone at the service, discuss how it works, and what options are available to you. The staff may give you a list of facilities for you to consider; you should visit them on your own and not simply take someone's word on how good they are.

2. Often some level of local government (city or town, region or county) has some responsibility for services to seniors in the community. In some cases they will run a long-term care setting (a nursing home, home for the aged, lodge), and provide services to seniors living at home. This government department may have a list of long-term care settings in the community that would be useful in starting your search. Be sure that the list contains not only those facilities that are run by the government, but also those operated by charitable non-profit groups such as a religious or ethnic organization, as well as those run privately.

    If your local government has not prepared such a list, check with the provincial government, or the Community Information Service in your community.

3. Recommendations from people who have had to seek long-term care settings for their family members can help you develop your list or narrow down the choices on a long list. However, it is important that you visit the recommended facilities, rather than simply taking someone else's word. Not only may there be differences in personal preferences, but facilities that are suitable for those who do not have Alzheimer Disease may not be equally suitable for those who do.

4. In some communities there are individuals or companies who help people find appropriate long-term care settings for their elderly family members for a fee. If you are considering using such a service, be sure to find out what they will do for you (give you a list, go to the facilities with you, help you fill out the applications) and what they estimate the costs will be. Most such services charge on an hourly basis.

WHAT TO LOOK FOR

Presented below is a check-list of things to look for when you are evaluating a facility. The check-list is only intended to serve as a guide, a list of things for you to think about. No setting will be perfect, and you will have to decide which features are most important. Facilities will vary on the extent to which they fit the criteria, and you should consider these items not just with a simple yes or no, but rather to what degree the setting fits with these criteria. You could rate each item by using a scale of one to ten to help yourself with the evaluation.

You may want to take this check-list with you when you visit a facility, and use it as a guide for your discussions with the administrator and staff. The written material the setting has sent you will also answer some of these questions. Some of them are things you will want to watch out for when you are taken on a tour of the setting.

While we will not comment here on all the items on the list, there are two that are important enough to require some extended discussion.

1. *Is there a separate unit for people with Alzheimer Disease and similar problems?* Many long-term care settings do not have separate units for people with Alzheimer Disease. We think this can be a major impediment to the quality of care a patient is likely to receive.

    Your experience as a caregiver has undoubtedly made you aware of the special adaptations that people with Alzheimer Disease require. They function best when the daily routine is clearly structured; when the physical environment is clear and unambiguous; and when the people who are providing their care have the patience and skills to help them function at the highest level of which they are capable.

    These circumstances are best achieved where people with Alzheimer Disease and similar disorders live together on a separate and special unit that accommodates their special circumstances. Just as it is unfair to expect older people who are mentally intact to understand and tolerate the difficult behaviours that are often found among people with Alzheimer Disease, so, too, it is unfair to expect people with Alzheimer Disease to function effectively in a unit with people who can maintain a faster and more complex pace of life.

2. *How well can the setting accommodate your family member when his or her condition deteriorates further?* The nature of Alzheimer Disease is such that a patient will continue to deteriorate after he or she has moved into the care setting. It is therefore important to pay attention to how the setting will accommodate increasing needs over time. Do they have units that provide higher levels of care than the one the patient would move into initially? Can they accommodate a bedfast patient or someone so frail as to be unable to move without help? When a patient becomes terminal, will they allow him or her to stay in the setting, or will they send the person to a hospital for terminal care?

While you may find it very difficult and painful to think about these kinds of issues, it is important to consider these factors in choosing a care setting for your family member. In the face of Alzheimer Disease one must plan for change, and failure to think about your family member's long-term needs, as well as the immediate needs, may lead to regret later on.

A CHECK-LIST[1]

1. *General Atmosphere* Who is responsible for the operation of the facility–a private owner, a religious or charitable organization, or the municipal government? Is the facility accredited by a recognized accreditation body? Is the home bright, clean, and decorated in a non-institutional manner? Do residents appear to be clean? Are they well groomed and appropriately dressed?

2. *Staff* Do staff smile, appear cheerful and show a positive attitude towards residents? Do staff treat residents, family, and other staff with dignity, courtesy, and respect? Do staff appear clean, neat and well-groomed? How willing are staff to spend time with you to answer your questions and talk about your needs and the needs of your family member? Are the staff who will be providing care to your family member specially trained to work with people with cognitive impairments?

3. *Foods and Beverages* Where do residents eat? Do they take their meals in a dining-room, or do they eat in a lounge, the corridor, or their bedrooms? Is the dining-room a pleasant place to eat? Is it attractively and appropriately decorated to look like a dining-room? How many residents eat together at one meal? Are residents given a choice of menu? (Ask to see a week's menu.) How does the food look and taste? (Try to get yourself invited to a meal.) Are guests allowed for meals? What provisions are made to assist residents who have difficulty eating on their own? Are family members allowed to come in and help to feed their resident? Are snacks served between meals? Are there facilities for family members to prepare a snack or a meal for their resident? Does the facility accommodate special diets? What are the policies about visitors bringing food for their family members?

4. *Bedrooms* How many residents share a bedroom? Are there provisions for privacy? In shared bedrooms, does each resident

[1]Adapted from The Council on Aging of Ottawa Carleton.

have private territory with a window or equal access to the window? Are residents permitted to bring any of their own furniture, subject to safety regulations? Are they permitted to bring other possessions, such as quilts, blankets, and afghans? Is there a place for residents to display small items such as knick-knacks and framed photographs? Is there a bulletin board for showing photographs and cards? Are residents permitted to hang pictures on the wall? Is there enough closet space? Where are out-of-season clothes stored? How is the lighting in the room? Do the windows provide for some natural light? Is there lighting near the resident's bed? Can lighting be individually controlled? How is the ventilation in the bedrooms? How is the temperature controlled? Do the windows open?

5. *Hygiene* Do the bedrooms contain an ensuite washroom? If not, how many residents share a washroom? Where are the washrooms located? Are there several toilets in one washroom? If so, what provision has been made for the privacy of residents while they are on the toilet? Is there a program to help reduce or prevent incontinence? How are residents cleaned after they have wet or soiled themselves? How frequently are residents bathed? Is there special equipment to help residents who have difficulty getting in and out of the bathtub? Is there a hairdresser or barber? What are the arrangements for personal laundry?

6. *Outdoor Areas* Are there interesting things for residents to see, do, and touch when they go outdoors? Are there outdoor activities programmed to encourage residents to go outdoors?

7. *Residents' Rights* What provisions have been made to allow you as a family member to express concerns on behalf of your resident?

8. *Visiting* What is the policy with respect to visiting? Are there special visiting hours, or can you come and go as you like? Are there places where you can visit with your family member in private? Are you permitted to take your family member out for a short time, such as a meal, a drive, or a family celebration? Where is the facility located? How easy is it for you to get there? Is there adequate parking, if you will be driving? Are there programs for family members and their residents to enjoy together?

9. *Activities* Is there an activities director? Is there a daily routine for residents to follow? Are there daily programs to keep residents busy? Are the programs designed for small groups? What is the staff to resident ratio in these programs? Are there opportunities for one-to-one contact between residents and staff? Are the programs and activities adapted to reflect the abilities of people with Alzheimer Disease? Are there opportunities for your family member to participate in activities of daily living, such as setting and clearing the table, drying dishes and putting them away, or small specific tasks related to meal preparation?

10. *Religion* Are there regular religious services in which your family member will be comfortable? Is there a religious environment with which you and your family member will be comfortable? Is there pastoral visitation?

11. *Language* What is the predominant language? Are services available in the first language of your family member?

12. *Financial* What are the financial arrangements? Are they clearly explained to you? Who sets the rates? How often do the rates change? How and when will you be billed? How does the facility look after a resident's money? Is there a trust account and does it pay interest? Is the resident charged for time spent in hospital? What is included in the standard charges? Are there extra charges for items such as laundry, activities, special equipment, cable T.V., hairdressing or barber, therapy, or specialized care such as dental care, foot care or incontinence care?

13. *Doctors* Are you permitted to continue using your family doctor? Who is the staff physician? How knowledgeable is he or she about aging, and about the special problems of people with Alzheimer Disease? How readily available is the staff physician? Is he or she on call twenty-four hours a day? How willing is the staff physician to spend time talking with family members? Will the staff physician consult with you about your family member's medical care? If your family member had to go to hospital, which hospital would he be taken to? Could the doctor who is looking after your family member in the facility (i.e., your family doctor or the staff physician) continue to look after your family member if he or she were admitted to hospital?

14. *Resident Care* How does the facility plan for individual preferences with regard to daily needs? Does the facility conduct comprehensive care planning conferences? Who attends these? Are family members invited to attend? Are there other opportunities for family members to have input into decisions about care for residents? Can residents receive specialized care, such as occupational therapy or physiotherapy? What is the facility's policy on physical and chemical restraints? Is it clearly written down and monitored? Are extraordinary measures used to sustain life? What is the position on DNR (Do Not Resuscitate) orders?

15. *Special Concerns for Alzheimer Patients* Is the layout of the unit designed to permit your family member to walk or pace if that is something he has been doing in the past? Does the design of the unit provide safety for residents who might wander away? Are the grounds designed so your family member can go outdoors at will, without your worrying that he may wander away?

VISITING FOR EVALUATION

The purpose of your visit is to evaluate the setting–to give you a sense of what it is like and how it operates. You may need more than one visit to accomplish this. Nevertheless, you should feel comfortable about visiting as often as necessary to ensure you have a clear picture on which to base your decision about whether you want your relative to live in the setting.

You should prepare for the visit by obtaining written information about the facility. You should specifically ask for information on their admission policies (who do they admit, what is the basis for deciding whether someone is appropriate for the facility) and application procedures.

Review the material and prepare a list of questions on details not covered in the written material, and on information that is confusing. You may want to use the check-list as a guide for preparing your questions, or even take a copy of the check-list with you when you make your visit.

For your first visit, you should meet with the person responsible for admissions. This will usually be the administrator or a staff person, such as a social worker or an admissions counsellor. During this initial meeting, you will probably want to accomplish three things: get an understanding of the admissions procedures; get an understanding of the way the facility is run, and how they deal with issues relating to care and quality of life for residents; take a tour of the setting. In addition to showing you what the setting looks like, the tour will give you a chance to see how the facility is run, how staff relate to the residents, and how care is provided.

If your family member has some special needs or preferences, ask how the facility will deal with them. Will they allow someone who is slow to get started in the morning to come to the dining-room in a bathrobe, and get dressed after breakfast? If music helps keep a patient calm, will they allow him or her to have ready access to music?

During the tour, you should feel free to ask questions about things you see and things you don't see. Sometimes in long-term care settings, and especially in units that provide care to Alzheimer patients things may not always be as they first seem. If something puzzles or surprises you, ask about it before you are too quick to make the wrong interpretation.

> The first time I visited the nursing home where my wife lives now I almost decided I'd never let her move there. I happened to be there at lunch, and I noticed a few residents eating in their rooms. I thought this was a terrible thing, and thought maybe they were being punished or something. Fortunately, I asked the nurse and she said these people had a lot of difficulty eating and were so easily distracted that it took forever for them to eat and their food got cold and then they didn't eat at all. So staff tried an experiment, and had them eat in their own rooms, at a table, and they did much better and ate more and seemed to enjoy the meals more. Staff spoke to their families, and everyone agreed this was a better solution than having these people eat in the dining-room and have to be fed by staff.

You may wish to visit more than once before you finally decide whether to apply to a particular facility. Visits to other settings you are considering may raise additional questions or you may simply wish to visit a setting again to make comparisons with other places easier.

Staff and administration at the facility should not object to a reasonable number of additional visits, or to your talking to staff members during those visits. However, you must balance your desire to get information from staff with an awareness that residents continue to require care.

PROFESSIONAL TECHNIQUES

During your visit to the care settings, and after your family member has moved in, you may hear staff talking about special approaches or techniques they use to relate to people with Alzheimer Disease and similar disorders. While it is not our intent to discuss these in any detail, a short description of some of the more commonly used terms may help you understand what staff are talking about.

Reality Orientation Reality orientation is an effort to keep people oriented to time, to place, and to who they are. Reality orientation is sometimes communicated through formal classes; however, we feel that the best reality orientation is for staff to incorporate it into the way they relate to residents on a twenty-four hour basis.

Validation Therapy Validation therapy is a technique developed by Naomi Feil in which the feelings of the confused person are validated in whatever time and place is real to him or her.

Motivation Therapy This therapy technique tries to restore the resident's interest in himself through specific structured sessions.

PREPARING FOR THE MOVE

You and your family member will have to prepare for the move, both physically and psychologically. The physical part of the move will be the easier. You will need to assemble and pack the things your family member will be taking along. This will be primarily clothing, and all of it will need to have the person's name in it. You should check with the administrator before putting name tapes in the clothing, because some places may want additional information in the clothing, such as the resident's room number or name of the building wing.

In addition to clothing, you should arrange to bring along some things that the patient is fond of, things that will make his or her room look more familiar and less institutional. This might be a favourite pillow, quilt or afghan; photos and pictures to hang on the wall; knick-knacks for a bookshelf or window-sill. It could even be a piece of furniture such as a favourite chair or a night-table, as long as it meets safety standards. Because things may get lost or damaged following the move, do not let a patient take anything that is very valuable.

You may be able to help prepare your family member for the move by having him or her visit the facility several times. While the patient probably will not remember the visit, the setting may seem somewhat familiar later. As well, these visits will give staff an opportunity to get to know your family member before the move.

It is probably not necessary or desirable to tell your family member about the move in advance. It is only likely to cause anxiety, and the person will likely forget anyway. On the day of the move, you should tell the patient that you are going to take him or her to another place to live where he will be safe and people will take very good care of him. Tell the patient that you will come to visit often. If the patient has been there before, you might remind him or her of the place and the people he or she has met there. In the first few days following the move, you should visit frequently to reassure your family member. A little photograph of yourself that the patient can keep nearby may also help relieve the initial anxieties.

If you think it will make it easier for you, ask another family member or a friend to come with you when you move your family member to the long-term setting. When the person is settled in, you and your companion may want to give yourselves a treat–lunch out, a movie, or a gift for yourself–to give yourself a reward for all the hard work you have done, including moving the patient. Alternatively, you may decide all you want to do is go home and have a good cry and a good sleep, and that makes sense too.

You will need to prepare yourself for the changes that will occur after your family member has moved. You will have more time and less responsibility than you have had in a long time. This may seem like a mixed blessing, as you suddenly find yourself alone with much more free time. Some caregivers immediately plunge back into the kind of lifestyle they had before they became a caregiver; others need time to regain their strength and energy, review their life, and think about what to do next.

Regardless of which type of person you are, plan to continue a consistent relationship with your family member after he or she has moved to another setting.

AFTER THE MOVE

Most family members like to continue helping with the care of a patient after he or she has been moved to a long-term care facility. In fact, the facility's attitude toward continued family involvement is sometimes a critical factor in deciding where to place a patient.

VISITING AND HELPING

Even though you care a great deal about your family member, visiting may be difficult after she or he has moved into the long-term care setting. This should not surprise you, if you think about how notoriously difficult it is to visit people who are in hospital–even when their mental faculties are fully operational.

There are, however, some ways to ease the strain of visiting your family member.

1. Many caregivers continue to function in that role by incorporating the provision of care into their visit. One of the most popular ways to combine visiting and caregiving is to help at mealtimes, which gives you an opportunity to visit the person while providing care and relieving the staff.

2. Some facilities schedule special events particularly for people with Alzheimer Disease and their families. In addition to helping you visit with your family member, they also provide an opportunity for you to meet the families of other residents in the unit.

    You may want to participate in support groups for families with relatives in the long-term care settings. Some facilities have special groups for families of Alzheimer patients. Participating in these groups will also help you get to know the families of other residents. As well, the groups provide an important source of advice and emotional support.

3. If there are programs elsewhere in the facility that your family member would especially enjoy, you might want to plan a visit around that. Your presence will ensure that the patient can attend, especially since the staff may not be willing to let her or him go alone.

My wife has always liked music, and it's been a source of real pleasure to her since she's been diagnosed as having Alzheimer Disease. I can't always go to the nursing home during the week to make sure she gets to the music programs, but every Sunday morning I go and take her to all the church services in the home, because she likes to listen to the hymns. She can't sing them anymore, but I always hold her hand, so she'll know I'm there, and sometimes when they're singing a hymn she'll give my hand a squeeze, or I'll feel her finger tapping a rhythm, and I know she's having a good time.

4. Sometimes a good visit means just sitting and holding your family member's hand. This is a way of letting the person know you are there, and that you care about him or her. If you do this in front of a television set, you may find the visit easier, and the patient may appreciate the normalcy of the two of you watching television together again.

5. There may be the opportunity for you and the patient to do something very simple together in the facility or on the grounds. Perhaps you will just go for a walk, or go to the cafeteria or snack bar for a cup of coffee.

HOW OFTEN SHALL I VISIT?

Obviously, there are no rules about how frequently you should visit your family member, except that you should visit as often as feels right. This may change over time, depending on the condition of the patient and your own needs. If your family member has moved to a long-term care facility to help relieve the burden on you, not much is gained if you place excessive demands on yourself with respect to visiting your family member.

When a patient has first moved to a long-term care setting, many people visit every day, or almost every day. This is not surprising, since you may want to feel assured that the person is receiving good care, and that the staff have all the information they need to help your family member function at the maximum level of ability.

After your family member has been living in the new facility for a while, you may discover that the frequency of your visiting has decreased. This is natural if you feel the person is receiving good care. With release from caregiving, you may find that there are new and interesting demands on your time: renewal of old friendships; or a return to a hobby or other activity that you gave up while you were providing care for your family member.

Eventually the patient will reach a stage where he or she does not know who you are, nor remember that you have been to visit recently. At this point, some caregivers feel it is no longer necessary to visit every day, though they do continue to visit as often as feels good for them.

FURTHER READING

Bausell, R. Barker, Rooney, Michael A. and Inlander, Charles B. *How to Evaluate and Select A Nursing Home.* Reading, Massachusetts: Addison-Wesley Publishing Company Inc., 1988.

Brown, Dorothy. *Handle with Care: A Question of Alzheimer's.* Buffalo, New York: Prometheus, 1984. (See "Nursing Homes: What to Look for," pp. 49-62.)

Thompson, Wendy. *Aging is a Family Affair: A Guide to Quality Visiting, Long-Term Care Facilities, and You.* Toronto: NC Press Limited, 1987.

APPENDIX

ALZHEIMER SOCIETIES

The following is a list of local chapters and provincial associations of Alzheimer Societies across Canada. This list was developed in February 1989 and current presidents of various chapters may not be the same. However, these people will be able to direct you to the appropriate contact person.

ALZHEIMER SOCIETY OF CANADA

Provincial Associations

British Columbia

Provincial Association
Marguerite Ford
Executive Director
Alzheimer Society of B.C.
#101 – 1090 West 8th Ave.
Vancouver, B.C.
V6H 1C4
(604) 736-0448

Box 1423, Stn. A
Kelowna, B.C.
V1H 7V8
(604) 768-2018

Prince George
Gladys Thorp, President
Alzheimer Society of
Prince George
P.O. Box 2864, Stn. B
Prince George, B.C.
V2N 4T7
(604) 564-6370

Kelowna
Marjorie Beals, President
Interior Alzheimer
Foundation

Powell River
Peter Newport, President
Alzheimer Society of
Powell River
R.R. #1, Reave Road
Powell River, B.C.
V8A 4Z2
(604) 487-9033

Alberta

Provincial Association
Jeanne Bentley, President
Alzheimer Association of
Alberta
1305 Centre Ave. N.E.
Calgary, Alta.
T2E 8K3
(403) 290-0110

Calgary
Greg Shyba, President
Alzheimer Society of Calgary
1305 Centre Ave. N.E.
Calgary, Alta.
T2E 8K3
(403) 290-0110 – Office

Camrose
Lloyd Reed, President
Alzheimer Society of Camrose
6202 – 49 Ave.
Camrose, Alta.
T4V 0P3
(403) 672-0021

Edmonton
Cully Wilson, President
Alzheimer Society of
Edmonton
1111 Jasper Ave., Rm. 8R-14
Edmonton, Alta.
T5J 1V1
(403) 429-4220

Grande Prairie
Mr. L. Larsen, President
Alzheimer Society of
Grande Prairie
Box 125
Grande Prairie, Alta.
T8V 3A1
Res. (403) 538-4151
Bus. (403) 539-2911

Lethbridge
Lily C. Rogers, President
Alzheimer Society of
Lethbridge and Area
1016 – 20th St. South
Lethbridge, Alta.
T1K 2C9
(403) 329-3766

Medicine Hat
Hope Johnson, President
Alzheimer Society of
Medicine Hat
P.O. Box 614
Redcliff, Alta.
T0J 2P0

Red Deer
Bob Johnstone, President
Alzheimer Society of
Red Deer
4512 Waskasoo Crescent
Red Deer, Alta.
T4N 2M2

Saskatchewan

Provincial Association
Shelly Wellar

Office Co-ordinator
S.A.R.D.A.
Regina General Hospital
1400 – 14th Avenue
Regina, Sask.
S4P 0W5
(306) 522-6881

Regina
Doris Balkwill, President
Alzheimer Society of Regina
2134 Winnipeg Street
Regina, Sask.
S4P 3X6
(306) 525-2154

Manitoba

Provincial Association
Barbara Wiktorowicz
Executive Director
Société Alzheimer Society of
Manitoba Inc.
205 Edmonton St.
Winnipeg, Man.
R3C 1R4
(204) 943-6622

Ontario

Provincial Association
Eileen Bigley
Executive Director
Alzheimer Association of
Ontario
131 Bloor St. West, Suite 423
Toronto, Ont.
M5S 1R1
(416) 967-5900

Barrie
Polly Denney, President
Alzheimer Society of Barrie

Box 1414
Barrie, Ont.
L4M 5R4
(705) 726-5889

Belleville/Hastings
Joy Dixon, President
Alzheimer Society of
Belleville/Hastings
R.R. #1
Plainfield, Ont.
K0K 2V0
(613) 477-2951

Brant
John Hart
Executive Director
Alzheimer Society of Brant
446 Grey Street, Suite 201
Brantford, Ont.
N3T 5V6
(519) 759-7692

Chatham–Kent
Jay Smith, President
Alzheimer Society of
Chatham–Kent
P.O. Box 182
Chatham, Ont.
N7M 5K3
(519) 692-4934

Cornwall
John Muir, President
Alzheimer Society of
Cornwall and District
P.O. Box 1852
Cornwall, Ont.
K6H 6N6
(613) 932-4914

Durham
Audrey MacLean, President
Alzheimer Society of Durham
40 King St. W., Suite 606
Oshawa, Ont.
L1H 1A4
(416) 576-2567

Grey-Bruce
Mabel Woodhouse, President
Alzheimer Society of
Grey-Bruce
757 2nd Avenue E.
Owen Sound, Ont.
N4K 2G9
(519) 376-7230

Guelph
Ardith Shipsides, President
Alzheimer Society of Guelph
Mailing – P.O. Box 213
Guelph, Ont.
N1H 6J9
Office – 70 Preston St.
Guelph, Ont.
N1H 3C4
(519) 836-7672

Haldimand-Norfolk
Mary Anne Baker, Chairperson
Alzheimer Society of
Haldimand – Norfolk
R.R. #1
Windham Centre, Ont.
N0A 1A0
(519) 426-7400

Halton/Wentworth
Georgia Wood, President
Alzheimer Society of
Halton/Wentworth

P.O. Box 36, Stn. "A"
Hamilton, Ont.
L8N 3A2
(416) 385-2142

Kingston
Kay McGeer, President
Alzheimer Society of Kingston
100 Stuart Street
Kingston, Ont.
K7L 2V6
(613) 544-3078

Kitchener/Waterloo
Jeff Sproat, President
Alzheimer Society of
Kitchener/Waterloo
40 Spadina Road West
Kitchener, Ont.
N2M 1E9
(519) 742-1422

Lambton
Annette Lawson, President
Alzheimer Society of Lambton
County
c/o Lambton Twilight Haven
R.R. #4
Petrolia, Ont.
N0N 1R0
(519) 882-1470

Leeds-Grenville
Ruth Lockett, President
Alzheimer Society of
Leeds-Grenville
P.O. Box 143
Maitland, Ont.
K0E 1P0
(613) 348-7106

London
Norma Nickle, President
Alzheimer Society of London
562 Wellington Street
London, Ont.
N6A 3R5
(519) 434-3138

Muskoka
Bill Adams, President
Alzheimer Society of Muskoka
Box 1483
Gravenhurst, Ont.
P0C 1G0
(705) 687-2769

Niagara Region
Sheila Nicholson, President
Alzheimer Society of
Niagara Region
5017 Victoria Ave.
Niagara Falls, Ont.
L2E 4C9
(416) 358-8151

North Bay
Murray Shave, President
Alzheimer Society of
North Bay
c/o Ms. Beth Campbell
Casselholme
400 Olive Street
North Bay, Ont.
P1B 6J4
(705) 474-4250

Northumberland
Marion Gellatly, President
Alzheimer Society of
Northumberland
Box 206

Port Hope, Ont.
L1A 3W3
(416) 885-5350

Orillia
Len Bull, President
Alzheimer Society of Orillia
P.O. Box 666
Orillia, Ont.
L3V 6K5
(705) 325-7233

Ottawa/Carleton
Kathy Wright
Executive Director
Alzheimer Society of
Ottawa/Carleton
Lower Level
1525 Carling
Ottawa, Ont.
K1Z 8R9
(613) 722-1424

Peel
Jim Fisher, President
Alzheimer Society of Peel
106 Lakeshore Rd., Suite 203
Mississauga, Ont.
L5G 1E3
(416) 278-3667 – 8:30–1:30

Peterborough
Bruce Found, President
Alzheimer Society of
Peterborough
Victoria & Haliburton
P.O. Box 1701
Peterborough, Ont.
K9J 7S4
(705) 748-5131 – office
(705) 742-2054 – res.

Porcupine
Monica Bevil, President
Alzheimer Society of
Porcupine District
694 Richelieu St.
Timmins, Ont.
P4N 5G6
(705) 267-1278

Prince Edward County
Joan Thissen, President
Alzheimer Society of
Prince Edward County
P.O. Box 980
Picton, Ont.
K0K 2T0
(613) 476-6872

Sault Ste. Marie & Algoma
Shelley McEachern, President
Alzheimer Society of
Sault Ste. Marie and
District of Algoma
316 Wellington St. W., Ste. 4
Sault Ste. Marie, Ont.
P6A 1J1
(705) 942-2195

Sudbury/Manitoulin
Otto Rennenkampff, President
Alzheimer Society for
Sudbury–Manitoulin District
970 Notre-Dame Avenue
Sudbury, Ont.
P3A 2T4
(705) 560-0603

Thunder Bay
Allison Smith, President
Alzheimer Society of Thunder
Bay
611 Sauier Street

Thunder Bay, Ont.
P7B 4A7
(807) 345-9556

Timmins
Monica Bevil, President
Alzheimer Society of
Timmins/Porcupine
P.O. Box 117
Timmins, Ont.
P4N 5G6
(705) 267-1278

Toronto
Daniel Andreae
Executive Director
Alzheimer Society for
Metro Toronto
21 Rippleton Rd.
Don Mills, Ont.
M3B 1H4
(416) 391-5300

Windsor/Essex
Don Fairley, President
Alzheimer Society of
Windsor/Essex County
1226 Ouellette Ave.
Windsor, Ont.
N8X 1J5
(519) 977-8911

York
Lorraine Inglis, President
Alzheimer Society of York
c/o Green Acres
194 Eagle Street
Newmarket, Ont.
L3Y 1J6
(416) 773-6404
Mon.–Wed.–Fri.

Québec

Provincial Association
M. Christian-Paul Gaudet
Président
La Fédération Québéçoise des
Sociétés Alzheimer
C.P. 325 Succursale E.
Montréal, P.Q.
H2T 3A8
(514) 731-3891

Laurentides
Réal Morin, Présidente
Société Alzheimer des
Laurentides Inc.
C.P. 276
Ste-Agathe-des-Monts, P.Q.
J8C 3A3
(819) 326-7136

L'Estrie
Lise Fèvre, Directrice
Société Alzheimer de l'Estrie
244, rue Dufferin, Local 260
C.P. 922
Sherbrooke, P.Q.
J1H 5L1
(819) 569-5262

Mauricie
Norman La Pointe, Président
Société Alzheimer de la
Mauricie
2541-A, boulevard de Carmel
Trois-Rivières, P.Q.
G8Z 3S3
(819) 376-7063

Montréal
Thelma Cadieux
Directeur Exécutif

Société Alzheimer de Montreal
3974, Notre-Dame Ouest
Montréal, P.Q.
H4C 1R1
(514) 931-4211

Outaouais
Yolande Gravel, Présidente
Société Alzheimer de
l'Outaouais
189, rue Magnus Ouest
Gatineau, P.Q.
J8P 2R3
(819) 663-3141 after 4:00
p.m.

Québec City
Janine Brosseau, Présidente
Société Alzheimer de Québec
3108, Chemin St-Foy
St-Foy, P.Q.
G1X 1P8
(418) 657-1880

Saguenay–Lac St-Jean
Noella Girard-Lalancette,
Présidente
Société Alzheimer de la
Sagamie
781 de la Lorraine Sud
Alma, P.Q.
G8B 2P2
(418) 668-7303

Sherbrooke
Josée Gosselih, Présidente
Société Alzheimer de l'Estrie
C.P. 922
Sherbrooke, P.Q.
J1H 5L1
(819) 569-5262

New Brunswick

Provincial Association
Carol Wyman, President
Alzheimer Society of New
Brunswick
P.O. Box 3327, Postal
Station B
Fredericton, N.B.
E3A 5H1
(506) 454-1969

Fredericton
Marsha Phelps, President
Alzheimer Society of
Fredericton
337 Canada St.
Fredericton, N.B.
E3A 4A3
(506) 472-5585

Saint John
Philip Francis, President
Alzheimer Society of
Saint John
26 Wasson Ct.
Saint John, N.B.
E2K 2K7
(506) 658-7191

Southeast New Brunswick
Evelyn Tetley, President
Alzheimer Society of
Southeast New Brunswick
P.O. Box 1266
Moncton, N.B.
E1C 8P9

Nova Scotia

Provincial Association
Paul McNair
Executive Director
Alzheimer Society of
Nova Scotia
Bayer's Rd. Shopping Centre
Starlight Gallery, Room 217
Halifax, N.S.
B3L 2C2
(902) 455-7347

Prince Edward Island

Provincial Association
Karen A. Clow, President
Alzheimer Society of P.E.I.
R.R. #2
N. Wiltshire, P.E.I.
C0A 1Y0
(902) 964-2780

Newfoundland

Provincial Association
Reginald Gabriel, President
Alzheimer Society of
St. John's (serving Nfld.)
c/o Leonard A. Miller Centre
100 Forest Road
St. John's, Nfld.
A1A 1E5
(709) 753-7736

SOCIAL SERVICES

Each province publishes a guide for services for seniors that you may obtain through your locally elected provincial representative or through the ministry in your province that publishes this document.

In addition, the federal government publishes a document called *Seniors' Guide to Federal Programs and Services* that can be obtained through your provincial Seniors Secretariat office. Other information or questions you may have can be answered through these offices. The addresses and phone numbers are shown below.

Federal Services Seniors
Secretariat in Ottawa
(613) 952-7358

British Columbia
Services to Seniors
848 Fort Street
Victoria, B.C.
B8W 3A1
(604) 682-0391
(604) 387-4331

Yukon
The Seniors' Information
Centre
3 – 106 Main Street
Whitehorse, Yukon
(403) 668-3383

Northwest Territories
Services for the Aged and
Handicapped
Northwest Territories
Department of Social Services
Yellowknife, N.W.T.
X1A 2L9
(403) 873-7276

Alberta
Senior Citizens Secretariat

Seventeenth Street Plaza,
Second Floor
10030 – 107 Street
Edmonton, Alta.
T5J 3E4
(403) 427-7876

Saskatchewan
Seniors Bureau
2151 Scarth Street, 1st Floor
Regina, Sask.
S4P 3Z3
(306) 787-7478

Manitoba
Manitoba Council on Aging
7th Floor
175 Hargrave Street
Winnipeg, Man.
R3C 3R8
(209) 945-3516

Ontario
Office for Senior Citizens'
Affairs
Queen's Park
76 College Street, 6th Floor
Toronto, Ont.
M7A 1N3
(416) 965-5106

Québec
Services des politiques et
plans socio-sanitaires
Ministère de la Santé et des
Services sociaux
1075, chemin Ste-Foy
4e étage
Québec, P.Q.
G1S 2M1
(418) 643-6024

New Brunswick
New Brunswick Senior
Citizens' Federation
Place Heritage Court
95 Foundry Street, Suite 421
Moncton, N.B.
E1C 5H7
(506) 857-8242

Nova Scotia
Nova Scotia Senior Citizens'
Secretariat
Dennis Building, 6th Floor
1740 Granville Street
Halifax, N.S.
B3J 1X5

or

Box 2065
Halifax, N.S.
B3J 2Z1
(902) 424-4737, 424-6322
1-800-424-0065

Prince Edward Island
Division of Aging and
Extended Care
Department of Health and
Social Services
P.O. Box 2000
Charlottetown, P.E.I.
C1A 7N8
(902) 368-4980

Newfoundland and Labrador
Division of Services to Senior
Citizens
Department of Health
P.O. Box 4750
St. John's, Nfld.
A1C 5T7
(709) 576-3551

LAWYER REFERRAL SERVICES

For legal questions, the Law Society of Canada has a helpful information number listed in your phone book. Look in the white pages under Law Society of Canada.

Because there are legal matters that you must deal with as a result of an Alzheimer patient's illness (Chapter 6), you will need a lawyer. Every lawyer in Canada must register with the Canadian Law Society, and each name is registered by the area and type of services the lawyer provides. Many provinces have a Lawyer Referral Service that you can call to ask for a referral in your area to deal with your circumstances.

Listed below are the cities that have Lawyer Referral Services. If your city is not listed, call the closest one for information on the entire province. If your province is not listed, you will have to call the Canadian Law Society.

Alberta
Calgary

British Columbia
Campbell River
Courtney
Cranbrook
Duncan
Kelowna
Naomi
Nelson
Prince George
South Caribou
Vancouver
Vernon
Victoria

Manitoba
Winnipeg

Nova Scotia
Dartmouth
Halifax

Ontario
Toronto

Quebec
Montreal

ACCOUNTANTS

If an Alzheimer patient has handled all of the financial matters in the past and it has become necessary for you to contact a chartered accountant, there are various ways to find one. Your first option may be to ask your lawyer or your bank manager for a recommendation. This is a usual procedure and is perfectly acceptable. You also may want to ask friends, family members, or the Alzheimer patient's previous business associates for suggestions. Another approach would be to call your Provincial Institute of Chartered Accountants (listed in the phone book) for a listing of accountants in your area.

UNDERSTANDING ALZHEIMER DISEASE: THE CAUSES AND POSSIBLE TREATMENTS

Donald R. McLachlan*

Everyone agrees that the cause of Alzheimer Disease remains unknown. Past experience with human disease teaches that without considerable understanding of the nature of underlying changes in the tissues affected by a disease, effective treatments or preventions cannot be developed. One of the mysteries about Alzheimer Disease is how an individual can have a normal, useful life and then develop the condition for no apparent reason. The fact that after the age of sixty the number of people with Alzheimer Disease doubles about every five years indicates that there must be something about the aging process itself that releases the condition. In brief, there is probably no single cause for Alzheimer Disease, but, rather, there are probably two sets of events that intersect to result in Alzheimer Disease: those events within the brain that occur during the normal process of aging and those events that are directly responsible for the disease. Therefore, both normal brain aging and the direct causes of Alzheimer Disease will have to be understood before we will be able to develop truly effective treatments.

Is Alzheimer Disease the result of inheritance or the result of something in the environment? Recently, a great deal of scientific activity has centred about the possible identification of inherited factors or genes

*Dr. McLachlan is professor of Medicine and Physiology and director of the Centre for Research in Neurodegenerative Diseases, University of Toronto.

for Alzheimer Disease. Although Alzheimer Disease is a common condition, some families appear more prone than others. Detailed study of such families sometimes indicates that the disease appears to be inherited as the result of a dominant gene that is not sex linked. In families in which the onset of illness occurs before the age of sixty, recent studies have shown that 50 percent of those individuals in the family will develop the disorder by the age of seventy-five. This pattern of inheritance indeed supports the idea that a dominant gene is responsible for the disease. In contrast, it has been shown that in families that exhibit late onset Alzheimer Disease (i.e., after the age of sixty), more than 50 percent of the family members develop the condition and indeed, of those family members who survive into the ninth decade, there may be up to 80 percent of them with the condition. This strongly argues against only a single dominant gene causing the disease and suggests that either there are multiple genes responsible or that the genetic background plus something from the environment must be important in the illness. However, it should be emphasized that both such type family inheritance patterns are rare.

Working with a small number of early onset families, Dr. Peter St. George Hyslop was able to demonstrate a linkage of the disease to a mutation that must lie in a specific region near the centre of chromosome 21. Chromosome 21 has long been suspected of carrying the gene for Alzheimer Disease because, in patients with Down's syndrome, Alzheimer Disease occurs at an unusually early age. Down's syndrome results from a genetic anomaly in which there are three, rather than two, copies of chromosome 21 in every body cell of the affected individual. In Down's Syndrome cases over the age of 40, virtually all individuals exhibit the brain changes of Alzheimer Disease. This has suggested that the extra gene copy or overworking of some region of the genes on chromosome 21 could cause Alzheimer Disease. It must, however, be noted that several laboratories working with other families, particularly those with late onset, are unable to demonstrate a linkage to chomosome 21. The current thinking is that there may be several gene loci that are responsible for the expression of Alzheimer Disease in those families that have a strong family history. Again it must be emphasized that such families as Dr. Hyslop has worked with are extremely rare, and a genetic factor probably is not important in more than 10 percent of all people who develop Alzheimer Disease. This means that something in the environment must be particularly important in causing the disease.

The strongest evidence suggesting that environmental factors are extremely important in the release of Alzheimer Disease comes from the study of identical twins. Identical twins carry exactly the same genetic inheritance patterns, and if a genetic factor were central to the release of the disease, then one would expect that both identical twins would develop Alzheimer Disease at about the same time in life. However, recent studies of identical twins have shown that only about 40 percent of such twins develop the disease concurrently and that 60 percent of identical twins may go ten, fifteen, or more years without developing the disease and die of other causes. Once again, this emphasizes that environmental factors are important.

From a therapeutic point of view, there is little we can do about our inheritance of genetic traits, but a search for and manipulation of environmental factors offers hope for treatment or prevention of Alzheimer Disease.

One approach to understanding Alzheimer Disease is to search for risk factors for the condition. Risk factors have been elucidated during epidemiological studies of the disease. Recently, Mortimer has reviewed those epidemiological studies in which information useful in assessing risk factors has been collected. As expected from the above discussion, a family history of Alzheimer Disease increases the odds ratio for developing the condition by a factor of 4, compared to individuals who do not have a family history. Interestingly, however, a prior head injury is also a significant factor for Alzheimer Disease and increases the risk approximately by three-fold. In terms of prevention, steps taken to prevent serious head injury during life are probably steps that could reduce the incidence of Alzheimer Disease.

It has also been known that aluminum in acidic drinking water may be a risk for Alzheimer Disease. Epidemiological studies in Norway and, more recently, in Britain indicate that the risk of developing Alzheimer Disease in areas with high aluminum-containing water is approximately 1.8 times greater than in geographic regions with low aluminum in the drinking water.

Another risk factor that does not quite reach statistical significance but for which there is a strong trend is thyroid gland dysfunction. Individuals who have a previous history of thyroid disease have a higher risk of developing Alzheimer Disease. Here the risk is about 1.5 times of those who do not have thyroid disease and suggests that understanding the causes of thyroid disease or the consequence of thyroid disease upon brain function may be very important in understanding the causes of Alzheimer Disease.

Unfortunately, other than these four risk ractors, no other environmental factors are known to be responsible or associated with Alzheimer Disease. While viruses have been investigated intensively for their possible role in this condition, no solid evidence indicates that the disease is transmissible or has any of the characteristics of any known transmissible disorder. However, it must not be forgotten that, after the First World War influenza epidemic, individuals who developed sleeping sickness many years later developed the histopathological changes associated with Alzheimer Disease, the neurofibrillary tangle in neurons in the brain stem. This delayed expression of one of the hallmarks of Alzheimer Disease, although associated more with Parkinsonism than with memory failure, continues to stimulate research into a possible delayed effect of viral infection. One of the future directions for research will be to carefully examine each of the risk factors that are now known for Alzheimer Disease and to search for additional risk factors that might be manipulated in the environment. Certainly, if aluminum is a risk factor for Alzheimer Disease, then human ingestion could be reduced, although the ubiquitous nature of aluminum would prevent total elimination from the environment.

Research into possible treatments for Alzheimer Disease has centred around the discovery that certain neurons that use certain chemicals for neurotransmission are selectively damaged. The most well-known group of neurons damaged in Alzheimer Disease are those that use acetylcholine as a neurotransmitter agent and whose cell bodies lie in the front regions of the brain. Damage to this particular group of neurons in the nucleus basalis results in memory difficulty in experimental animals, and memory improvement can be achieved by either replacing the acetylcholine deficit with a chemotherapeutic agent or implanting into the damaged region acetylcholine-containing fetal cells. Clinical trials with acetylcholine replacement in Alzheimer patients, however, have failed to indicate that a useful therapeutic benefit can result from this approach. Many investigators feel that failure to treat patients with Alzheimer Disease based on neurotransmitter replacement has occurred because the acetylcholine cells are not the only neurons to be damaged in Alzheimer Disease and that design of an appropriate mixture of neurotransmitter agents might be more helpful. It is known that several neurotransmitter deficits occur in this disease and replacement therapy might be designed along these lines. Unfortunately, trials based on these concepts have been few in number and the results do not indicate a positive benefit to the patient or the family.

While research into implantation of healthy brain cells into a damaged human brain holds some promise, it is questionable whether this technique will ever be useful in Alzheimer Disease since the disease is associated with widespread damage in the brain involving the cerebral cortex and many subcortical structures. This means that the anatomical distance between regions is so great that the simple implantation of healthy tissue is unlikely to be able to ever make adequate contacts to establish normal function. Thus it is unlikely that brain transplants will have a useful role in this particular condition.

Perhaps the more useful therapeutic approach would come from a precise understanding of the essential lesions or disorders associated with Alzheimer Disease. These essential changes appear to occur at two levels: the level at which the insult kills neurons and the level at which neurons become nonfunctional but still survive. There are those workers who believe that it is neuron death that is the determinant of the clinical difficulties that an individual with Alzheimer Disease exhibits. If this latter idea is correct, then the underlying mechanism that kills the neuron is of paramount importance. At the present time, there are several candidates that do offer some therapeutic intervention. For instance, there is some evidence that free radicals that form during normal brain metabolism are improperly handled by the Alzheimer brain and that this factor may damage the membranes resulting in cell death. If so, clinical trials based on ways to deal with free radical control may hold some promise for the future treatment of Alzheimer Disease. It is also known that neurons require high fluxes of calcium across their membranes in order to carry on normal function. However, when calcium fluxes are not properly buffered intracellularly, the calcium ion can release destructive enzymes that attack essential structures within the neuron, resulting in neuron death. Regulation of calcium flux has become an important adjunct to the treatment of acute heart attacks, and the possibility of applying this understanding to the prevention of further neuron death in Alzheimer Disease is certainly justified. It is also known that neurons release certain amino acids, such as glutamic and aspartic acid, and these excitatory amino acids can become toxic when the flux of calcium is greater than the buffering capacity of the neuron. It appears that Alzheimer Disease is concerned with the loss or down regulation of the proteins that buffer calcium, and, again, methods to control both the calcium flux and the excitatory toxic amino acids may offer some future direction for the treatment of Alzheimer Disease.

Finally, it is known that certain chemicals and plant substances may be toxic to the central nervous system and may induce delayed neuron death. On the Island of Guam it has been speculated that a toxic amino acid, which occurs in one of the natural occurring plants used for the preparation of flour, may be toxic to the nervous system when ingested. A detailed study of this amino acid is underway at present in a number of laboratories and emphasizes that research will have to be done into a variety of foodstuffs and environmental contaminants that may have delayed effects upon the nervous sytem.

While this discussion may appear to indicate that a treatment or prevention is far over the horizon, it must be emphasized that the tools available to the investigator of Alzheimer Disease are far more sophisticated today than they have ever been. These tools are extremely powerful in understanding how the neurons become altered in their function and offer much more hope for the future than might be suspected from past experience.

Alzheimer Disease, like all serious illnesses for which no effective treatment is available, encourages individuals to seek unconventional treatments. In today's medical and scientific community, every effort is being made to produce an effective, safe treatment. It is important that therapeutic trials be undertaken, but it is strongly recommended that a family contemplating such a trial be assured that the therapeutic trial is being conducted by an established and reputable research team and that the procedures have been reviewed by an ethics committee to assure that the best interests of the Alzheimer patient are being considered.